COLOUR GUIDE

PICTURE T

CW00548465

Clinical M

Peter C. Hayes MD PhD FRCP (Edin)

Senior Lecturer in Medicine
Department of Medicine and Centre for Liver and Digestive Disorders
Royal Infirmary
Edinburgh

Niall D. C. Finlayson PhD FRCP (Edin)

Consultant Physician
Centre for Liver and Digestive Disorders
Royal Infirmary
Edinburgh

Churchill Livingstone

EDINBURGH LONDON MADRID MELBOURNE NEW YORK AND TOKYO 1994

CHURCHILL LIVINGSTONE
Medical Division of Longman Group Limited

Distributed in the United States of America by
Churchill Livingstone Inc., 650 Avenue of the Americas,
New York, N.Y. 10011 and by associated companies,
branches and representatives throughout the world.

First published 1994
  Reprinted 1995

ISBN 0–443–04957–2

British Library Cataloguing in Publication Data
A catalogue record for this book is available from the
British Library.

Library of Congress Cataloging in Publication Data
A catalogue record for this book is available from the
Library of Congress.

For Churchill Livingstone

Publisher
Laurence Hunter
Project Editor
Jim Killgore
Editor
Adele Mighton
Production
Nancy Arnott
Design Direction
Judith Wright
Sales Promotion Executive
Marion Pollock

The
publisher's
policy is to use
**paper manufactured
from sustainable forests**

Printed in Hong Kong
GC/02

Preface

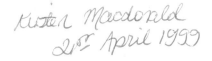

In everyday clinical medicine, as well as in examinations, physical signs arise that require explanation. Although there are many books illustrating numerous physical signs accompanied by background text the aim of this book is to stimulate both recognition and interpretation. This approach we hope will help students both integrate their knowledge of medicine as a whole, when it is so often compartmentalized, and prepare for examinations.

We are grateful to all the authors of Churchill Livingstone books who have allowed us to use their illustrations.

Edinburgh   P.C.H.
1994   N.D.C.F.

Acknowledgements

Most of the illustrations used in this book have appeared in other volumes in the Colour Aids and Colour Guides series. The publishers and authors kindly acknowledge the following for their permission to re-use existing photographs or for providing new examples.

Dr J L Anderton
Dr A P Ball
Dr D Bell
Mr M A Birchall
Dr M Crockford
Dr T W Evans
Dr D A Fenton
Dr J A Gray
Dr G Holdstock
Mr G Hooper
Mr J J Kanski
Professor C Kennard
Mr D W Lamb
Professor D Linch

Dr A McMillan
Dr J M H Moll
Dr S M Murphy
Dr G R Scott
Dr S Shaw
Mr N D Stafford
Dr M Swash
Dr D Thomson
Dr P Trend
Dr J D Wilkinson
Dr P H Wise
Mr A P Yates
Mr R Youngs

The illustrations have been taken from the following volumes in the Colour Aids and Colour Guides series: Chest Medicine; Clinical Signs; Dermatology; Endocrinology; ENT; Gastroenterology and Liver Disease; Haematology; Hand Conditions; HIV Infection and AIDS; Infectious Diseases; Nephrology; Neurology; Ophthalmology; Orthopaedics; Rheumatology and Sexually Transmitted Diseases.

Contents

Questions

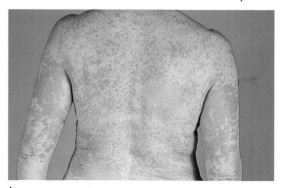

1. This 47-year-old man was being treated for acute bronchitis by his own doctor. He then presented to casualty with the appearance illustrated.
a. What abnormality is shown?
b. What is the likely underlying cause?

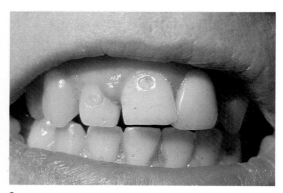

2. These abnormalities occurred in a patient with epilepsy.
a. What abnormalities are shown?
b. What may be the underlying condition?

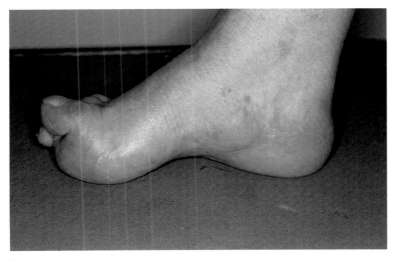

3. This 10-year-old girl had weakness of her calf muscles and loss of ankle jerk reflexes. Diminished vibration sense was found below the knee.
a. What is the likely underlying diagnosis?
b. How is it inherited?

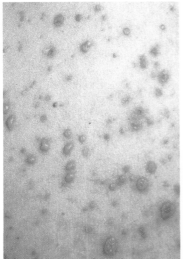

4. Crops of these lesions appeared on the axial parts of this patients body.
a. What lesions are present?
b. What is the disorder?

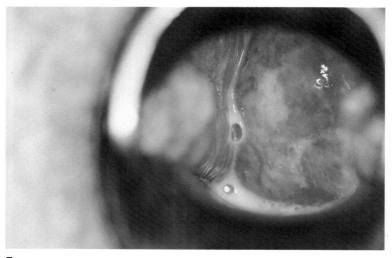

5. This 26-year-old woman complained of vaginal discharge, dyspareunia and dysuria.
a. What is the likely diagnosis?
b. How should it be treated?

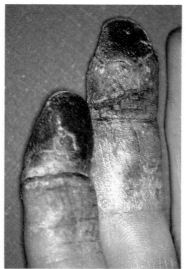

6.
a. What condition is illustrated here?
b. List three disposing causes.

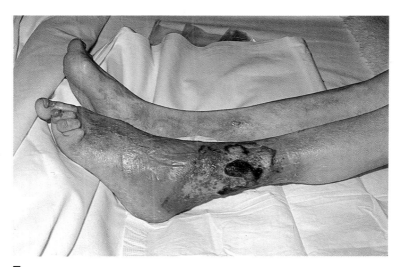

7. **This 65-year-old lady with a long history of rheumatoid arthritis was found to have an enlarged spleen.**
a. What two abnormalities are illustrated in this figure?
b. What is the likely syndrome?

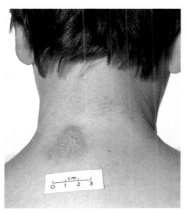

8. **A 19-year-old man complained of photophobia, malaise and neck stiffness.**
a. What abnormality is shown?
b. What is the likely cause of his symptoms?
c. How should this be treated?

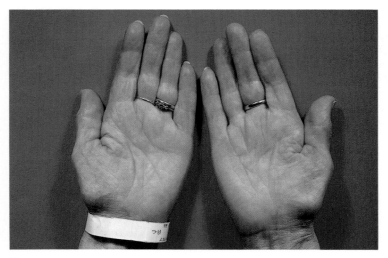

9. This 57-year-old woman complained to her general
practitioner of tingling in her hands especially at night.
a. What physical sign is present?
b. What is the likely underlying cause?

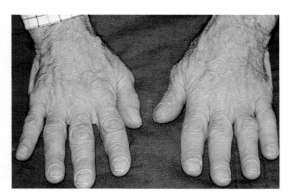

10. This 67-year-old man originally presented to his dentist
with jaw pain. He also complained of headaches and episodes
of severe sweating.
a. What is the likely diagnosis?
b. What other signs should be sought?

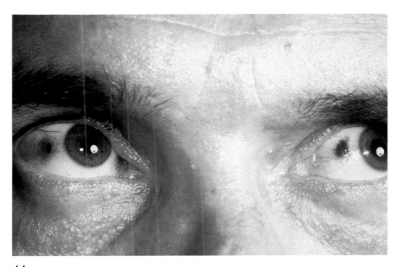

11. **This 37-year-old man complained of a long history of knee, shoulder and hip pain.**
a. What abnormality is shown?
b. What is the likely underlying diagnosis?

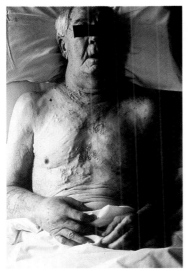

12. **This 71-year-old man was admitted with breathlessness and haemoptysis.**
a. What is the diagnosis?
b. What early treatment should be considered?

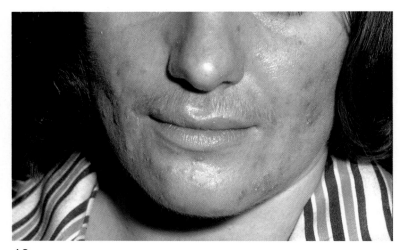

13. This 19-year-old woman complained to her general practitioner of oligomenorrhoea.
a. What is the probable diagnosis?
b. What is the differential diagnosis?

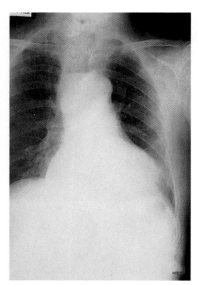

14. This 61-year-old woman complained of dysphagia for 2 years.
a. What 2 abnormalities are shown in this X-ray?
b. How should the underlying disorder be treated?

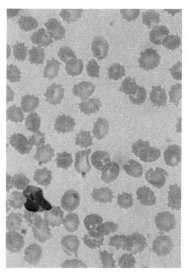

15.
a. What abnormality is shown on this blood film?
b. With what conditions is it associated?

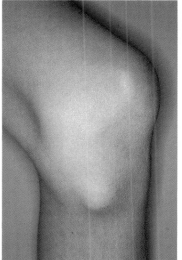

16.
a. What is the likely diagnosis?
b. How should it be treated?

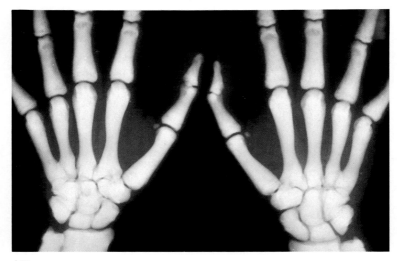

17. **This patient was suffering from anaemia.**
a. What diagnosis is shown in this photograph?
b. What other complication had arisen recurrently in previous years?

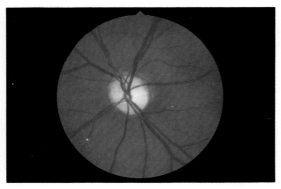

18.
a. What abnormality is illustrated?
b. List four causes.

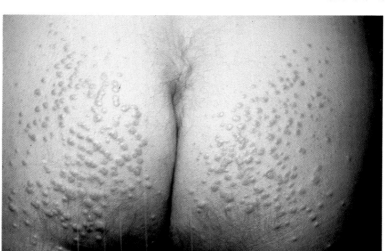

19. These lesions arose in a patient with newly diagnosed diabetes mellitus.
a. What abnormality is shown?
b. How should it be treated?

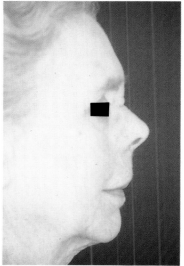

20. This lady was complaining of cough and haemoptysis.
a. What is the likely underlying diagnosis?
b. What investigations should be undertaken?

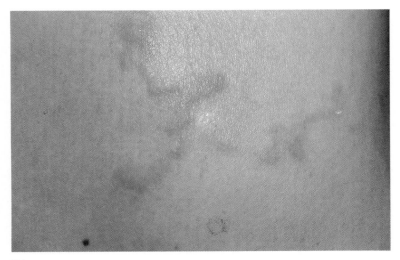

21. This itching lesion appeared in a patient travelling in South America.
a. What is the lesion called?
b. What part of the body was most likely involved?
c. Name one possible cause.

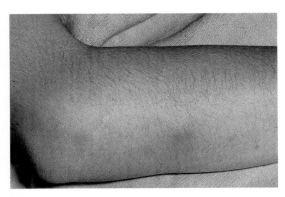

22. A 36-year-old woman presented with an acutely painful elbow. She was found to have a high ESR and an increased serum calcium.
a. What two abnormalities are illustrated in this picture?
b. What diagnosis should be considered and what investigations are appropriate?

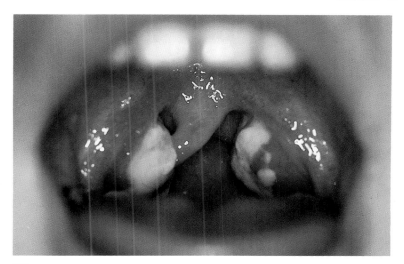

23. This 17-year-old girl was generally unwell and complained of a sore throat. She was mildly icteric and liver function tests showed hepatitic abnormalities.
a. What is the diagnosis?
b. What two other abnormalities may be found on examination?

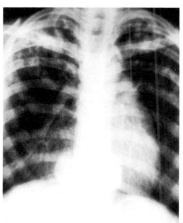

24. This is the chest X-ray of a patient with weight loss and fever.
a. What abnormality is shown?
b. What investigations should be undertaken?

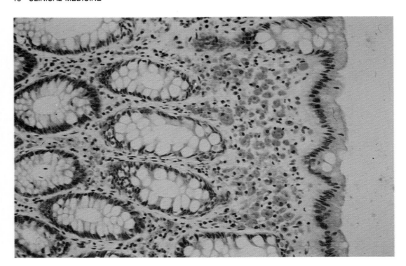

25. This biopsy was obtained from a middle-aged lady complaining of persistent constipation.
a. What abnormality is shown?
b. What is the likely underlying cause?

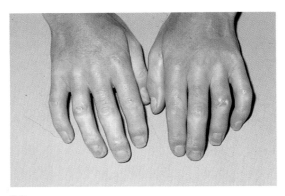

26.
a. What abnormality is illustrated?
b. What is its significance?

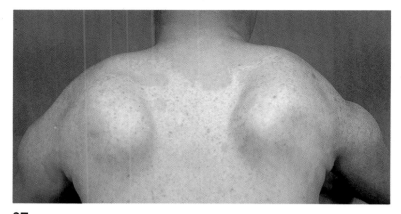

27. This 15-year-old boy presented with upper limb weakness.
a. What abnormalities are illustrated?
b. What is the likely underlying cause?

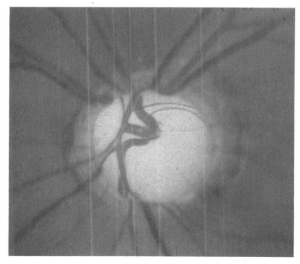

28. Fundoscopy showed this appearance in an asymptomatic 62-year-old man during an employment-related examination.
a. What abnormality is shown?
b. What investigation would reveal abnormalities caused by this lesion?

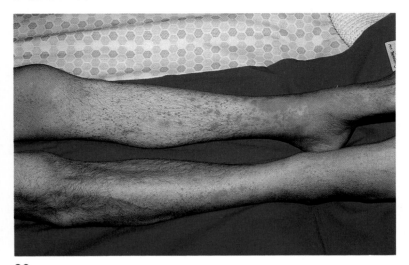

29. A 45-year-old man with ulcerative colitis presented with haematuria.
a. What abnormality is illustrated?
b. What might it be due to?

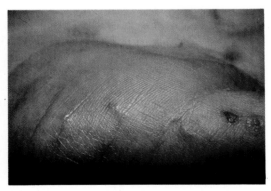

30. This 26-year-old boarding school boy complained of itchy hands in bed at night.
a. What abnormality is shown?
b. What is the underlying cause?

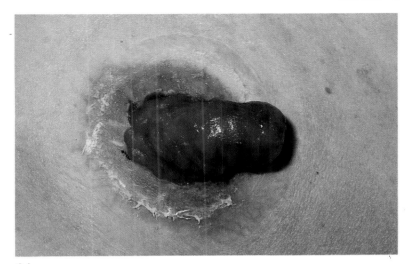

31. A 48-year-old lady had sclerosing cholangitis and a previous colectomy for ulcerative colitis. She complained that the ileostomy bag had suddenly filled with blood.
a. What was the bleeding due to?
b. How should it be treated?

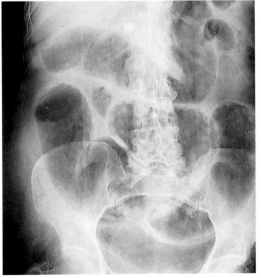

32. A 71-year-old man presented with abdominal pain and diarrhoea.
a. What abnormality is shown?
b. What is the underlying cause?

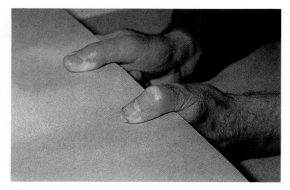

33.
a. What clinical sign is illustrated here?
b. Of what is it diagnostic?

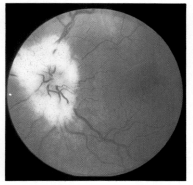

34.
a. What abnormality is shown here?
b. With what may it be confused?
c. What visual deficiency does it cause?

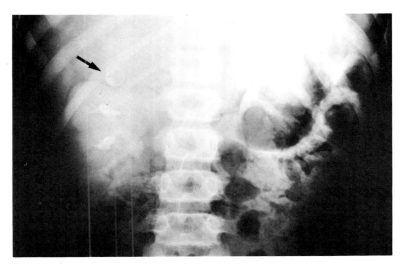

35.

a. What is illustrated in this abdominal X-ray?

b. What may be the underlying pathology?

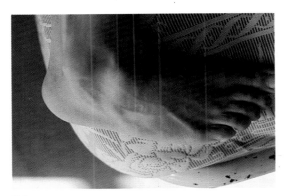

36. This photograph is of the lateral side of a foot of patient with pes cavus.

a. What abnormality is shown?

b. What is the likely diagnosis?

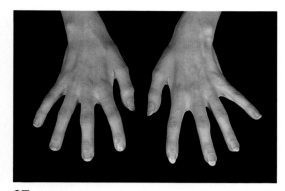

37. A 48-year-old woman complained of progressive weakness over some months and recently difficulty in swallowing and speaking.
a. What abnormality is present?
b. What is the underlying diagnosis?

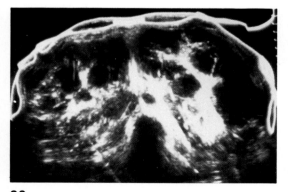

38. A 36-year-old man with hypertension and haematuria had this ultrasound examination.
a. What abnormality is illustrated?
b. Name a vascular lesion with which this disease is associated.

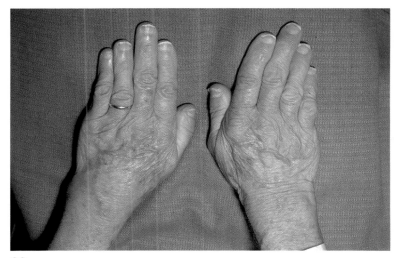

39.
a. What abnormality is shown in this figure?
b. What may be the underlying cause?

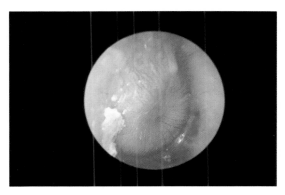

40. A 6-year-old boy was referred because his speech was developing slowly and his performance at school was poor. Otoscopy was carried out.
a. What abnormality is present?
b. What is the most likely underlying cause?

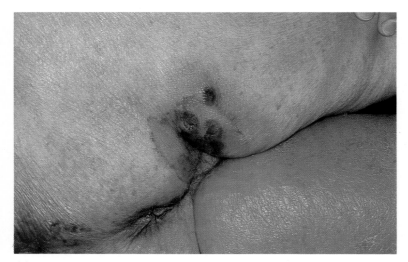

41. A 46-year-old lady with a long history of arthralgia and recent weight loss showed these signs on examination.
a. What is the lesion shown?
b. What is the likely underlying diagnosis?

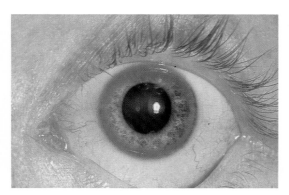

42. This 22-year-old girl complained of lethargy and was found to have anaemia and abnormal liver function tests.
a. What is the abnormality shown?
b. Name two further investigations which would confirm the diagnosis.

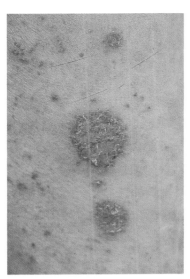

43. This 45-year-old business executive complained of this intensely pruritic eruption.
a. What condition is shown?
b. What aetiological factors may be involved?

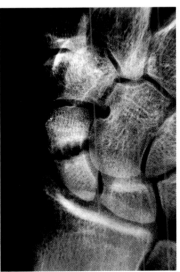

44. A 42-year-old man complained of a painful wrist after falling whilst skiing.
a. What abnormality is shown?
b. How should it be treated?

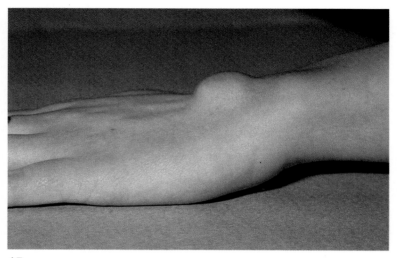

45. A 26-year-old lady was found to have this abnormality incidentally at antenatal screening.
a. What is the likely diagnosis?
b. How should it be treated?

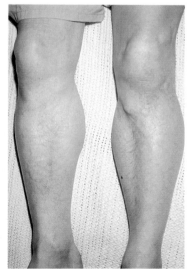

46. This patient presented with rectal bleeding.
a. What abnormalities are shown?
b. What is the underlying syndrome called?

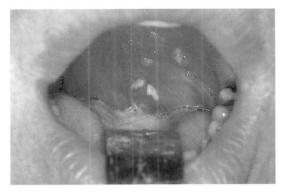

47. A 16-year-old boy complained of a holiday illness with fever, malaise and an increasingly sore throat; the pain prevented him swallowing his saliva. A clinical examination revealed cervical lymphadenopathy.
a. What abnormality is illustrated?
b. How should this be treated?

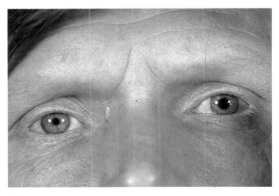

48. A 21-year-old woman was found on medical examination to have an enlarged left pupil which showed no light reaction.
a. What is the diagnosis?
b. What is its significance and what other neurological feature may be found?

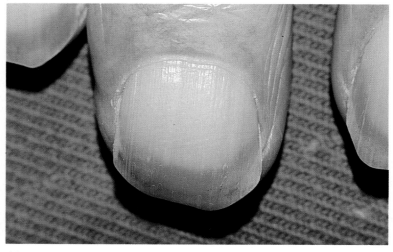

49.
a. What physical sign is illustrated?
b. What is its significance?

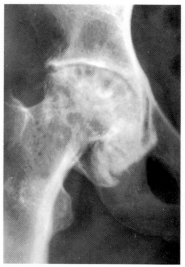

50. This 73-year-old lady presented with progressive pain, particularly in the evenings, in her right hip.
a. What is the diagnosis?
b. How should it be treated?

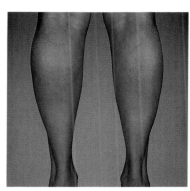

51. This patient has difficulty walking.
a. What abnormality is shown?
b. What is the the underlying disease?

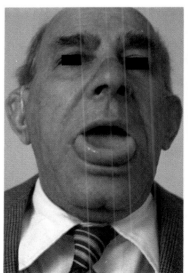

52. This patient presented with increasing tiredness and was found to have proteinuria.
a. What does this figure demonstrate?
b. What may be the underlying cause?
c. How do you confirm the diagnosis?

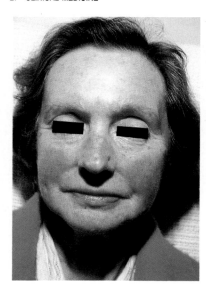

53. **This 67-year-old lady was complaining of diarrhoea, abdominal cramps and wheeze.**
a. What physical sign is shown?
b. What is the most likely finding on abdominal examination?
c. What one investigation would you do?

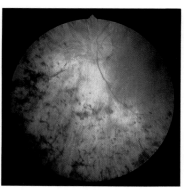

54.
a. What is this condition?
b. With what conditions may it be associated?

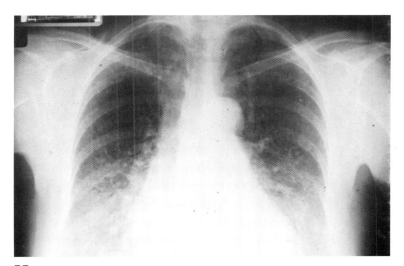

55. This patient complained of recurrent haemoptysis and had an increased pulmonary CO diffusing capacity.
a. What is the abnormality shown?

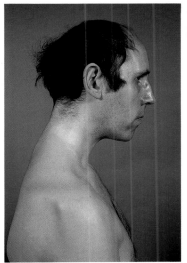

56.
a. What is the diagnosis?
b. What features are associated with this condition?

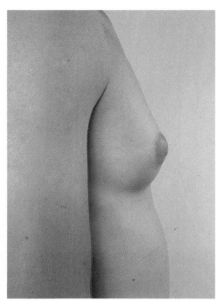

57. A 51-year-old man under investigation for breathlessness, complained of sudden onset of pain in the right breast.
a. What abnormality is shown?
b. What is the likely underlying cause?
c. How should this be confirmed?

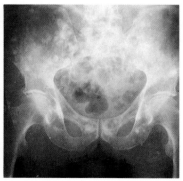

58. This is a pelvic X-ray of a 71-year-old man with a short history of nocturia and haematuria.
a. What abnormality is present?
b. What underlying diagnosis should be considered?

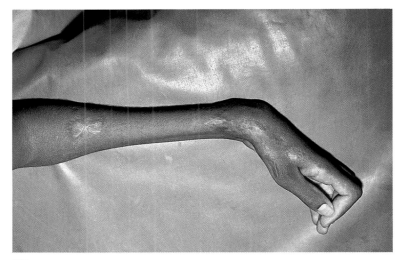

59.

a. What is the likely diagnosis illustrated here?
b. What is the probable predisposing cause?

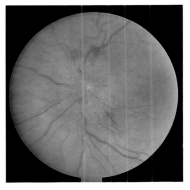

60.

a. What is this abnormality?
b. Give two possible underlying causes.

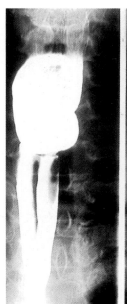 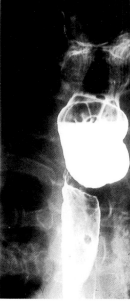

61.

a. What abnormality is shown?

b. Name two complications which may arise.

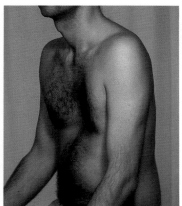

62. This 37-year-old man was undergoing an insurance medical examination.

a. What abnormality is noted?

b. What is its significance?

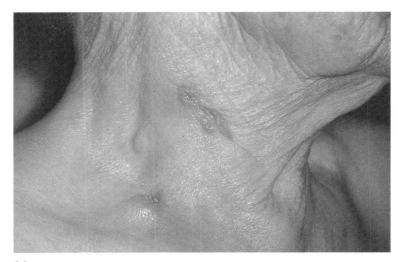

63. This elderly lady presented with weight loss and cough.
a. What is the abnormality shown?
b. How should the cause be identified?

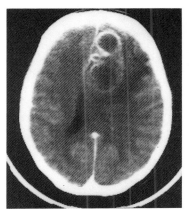

64. This 71-year-old man presented to casualty after having an epileptic fit.
a. What abnormality is shown on this CT scan?
b. What are the predisposing causes?

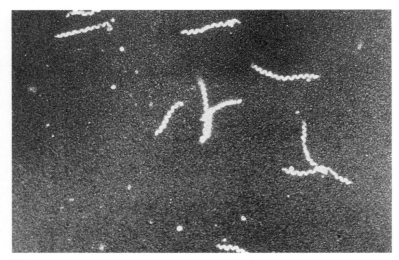

65.
a. What investigation is shown here?
b. What further tests should be undertaken to confirm the diagnosis?

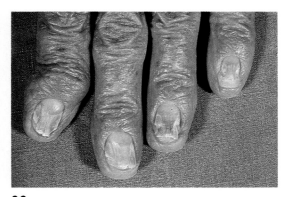

66. This man presented with severe diarrhoea. He had alopecia and investigation showed intestinal polyps.
a. What abnormalities are shown?
b. What is the syndrome?

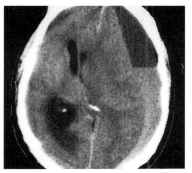

67. A 57-year-old man known to abuse alcohol was admitted to Accident & Emergency confused and with a mild right hemiparesis.
a. What abnormality is shown?
b. How should it be treated?

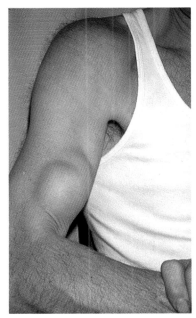

68. A 55-year-old man complained of a lump in his right arm but was otherwise asymptomatic.
a. What is the diagnosis?
b. How should it be treated?

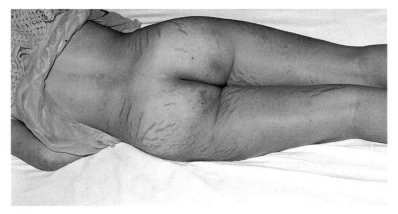

69.
a. What medical sign is illustrated here?
b. What is the most likely cause?

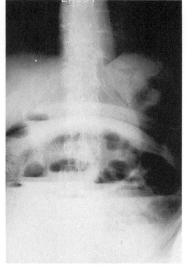

70. A 36-year-old man was seen in Accident & Emergency with nausea, anorexia and vomiting.
a. What does the erect film demonstrate?
b. What does this sign indicate?

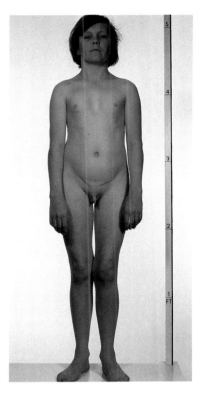

71. This young man complained of anosmia.
a. What features are illustrated?
b. What may be the underlying syndrome?

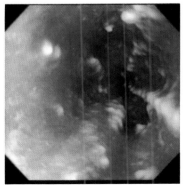

72. A 44-year-old ex intravenous drug abuser who was known to have had hepatitis B 15 years before was undergoing investigation for weight loss.
a. What two abnormalities are shown here?
b. What further investigation should be considered?

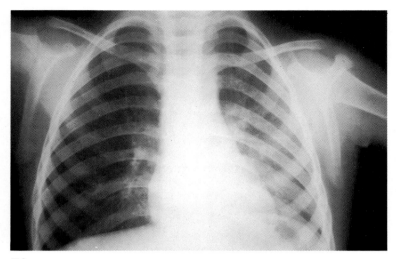

73. An 11-year-old child complained of breathlessness on the night following a childrens' party.
a. What abnormality is shown?
b. What is the probable cause?

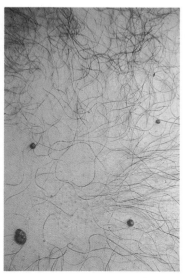

74. This 67-year-old man complained to his general practitioner of spots on his abdomen.
a. What abnormality is illustrated here?
b. What is their significance?

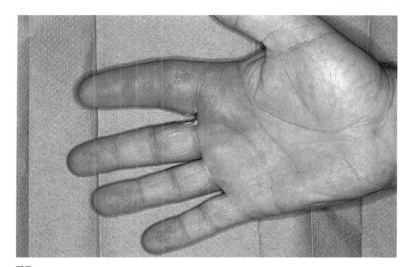

75. **This 32-year-old man complained of a painful hand three days after a brawl in a public house in which he thinks his hand was bitten.**
a. What abnormality is shown?
b. How should it be treated?

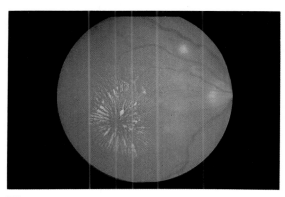

76.
a. What abnormalities are shown here?
b. What is the probable underlying cause?

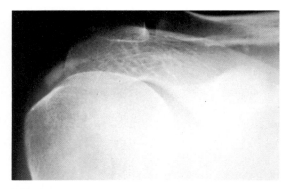

77. **This 45-year-old lady complained of pain of sudden onset in her right shoulder which was hot and tender on examination.**
a. What is the diagnosis?
b. How should it be treated?

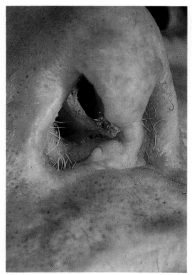

78. **This 63-year-old destitute man had lived in a hostel for 10 years.**
a. What condition is illustrated?
b. How should it be treated?

79.
a. What two abnormalities are shown in this picture?
b. What is the reason for the linear lesion?

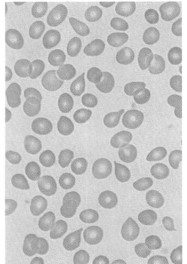

80. A 68-year-old lady with anaemia and splenomegaly had this blood film.
a. What does it show?
b. What is the likely underlying diagnosis?

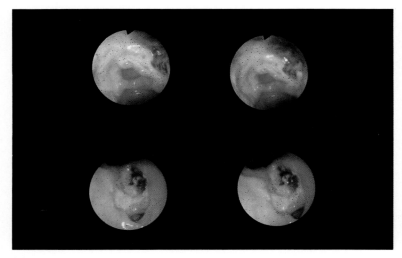

81. **This 61-year-old lady with rheumatoid arthritis taking non-steroidal anti-inflammatory drugs presented with falling attacks.**
a. What abnormality is illustrated?
b. How should it be treated?

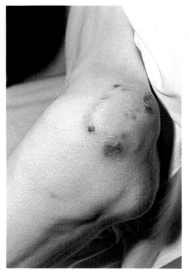

82.
a. What abnormality is illustrated?
b. What is its clinical significance?

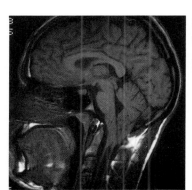

83.
a. What abnormality is illustrated in this MRI scan?
b. To what condition does it predispose?

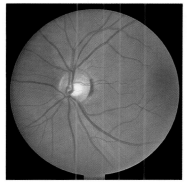

84. This man underwent a routine medical examination.
a. What comment would you make?

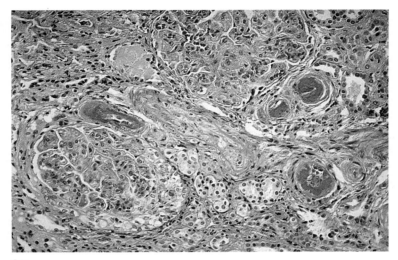

85. A 37-year-old man presented with sudden hemiplegia. He was found to have renal failure.

a. What abnormality is shown in his renal biopsy?
b. What two features might be seen on fundoscopy?

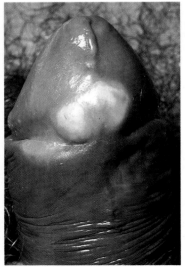

86.

a. What does this demonstrate?
b. What is the causative organism?
c. What is the most common complication in this condition?

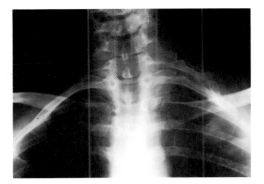

87. A 35-year-old man complained of shooting pains in his left arm with paraesthesia and numbness.
a. What abnormality is shown?
b. What further investigations should be undertaken?

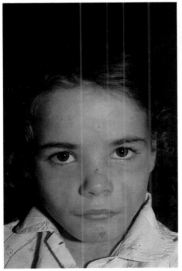

88. This 12-year-old girl was admitted with fever, tachycardia and arthralgia.
a. What physical sign is shown?
b. What is the underlying cause?

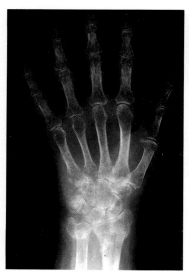

89. A 27-year-old man with a past history of a road traffic accident complained of a painful left hand.
a. What is the diagnosis?
b. What is the cause in this case?

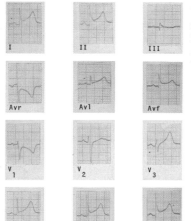

90. This ECG was obtained from a 48-year-old man who had chronic renal failure.
a. What does it show?
b. What is the probable cause?

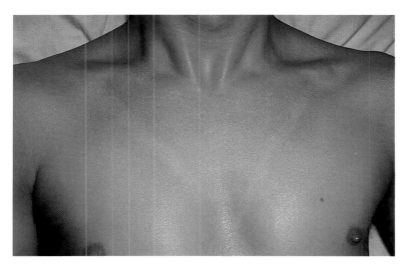

91. This feature was found at a routine pre-employment examination.
a. What physical sign is demonstrated here?
b. What is its significance?

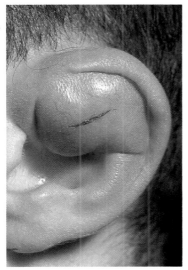

92.
a. What abnormality is shown?
b. How should it be treated?

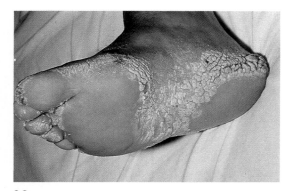

93. This patient had diarrhoea and ankle pain.
a. What abnormality does the foot show?
b. What is the underlying syndrome? Name one other systemic manifestation of this syndrome.

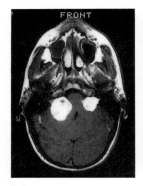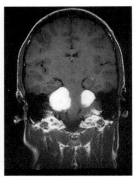

94. A 42-year-old man complained of progressive deafness, tinnitus and facial pain.
a. What abnormality is shown?
b. What is the likely diagnosis?
c. What underlying condition may be present?

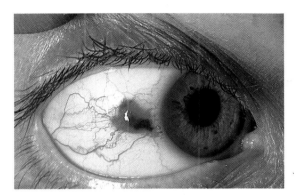

95. What abnormality is shown in this slide?

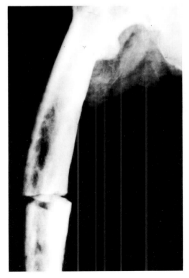

96. This 65-year-old woman presented with a fracture of her femur.

a. What is the cause of the fracture shown in the X-ray?
b. What biochemical abnormality is found in the blood?
c. What complications may arise?

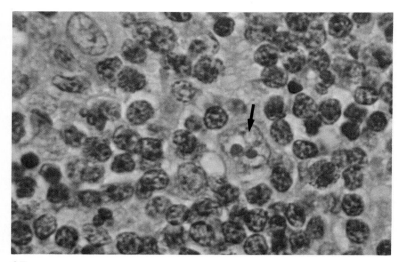

97. **A 25-year-old man presented with night sweats and cervical lymphadenopathy. Biopsy of the node was undertaken.**
a. What abnormality is shown (arrowed)?
b. What is the underlying diagnosis?

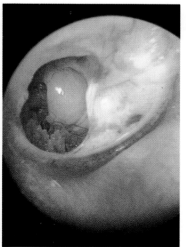

98. **A 16-year-old boy complained of ear discharge and deafness.**
a. What abnormality is shown?
b. How should it be treated?

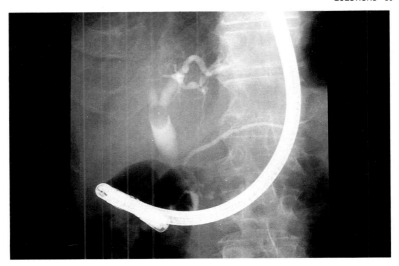

99.
a. What investigation is shown here?
b. What abnormality is present?
c. How should it be treated?

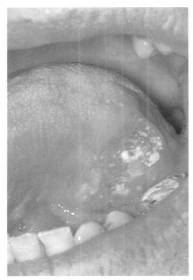

100.
a. What abnormality is shown here?
b. How should it be confirmed?

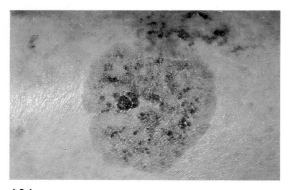

101. This abnormality occurred on the upper thigh.
a. What is it?
b. With what may it be associated?

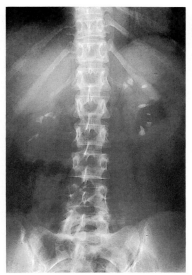

102. A 48-year-old Australian lady who worked as a typist complained of haematuria and polyuria.
a. What abnormality is illustrated in this abdominal film?
b. What is the likely cause?

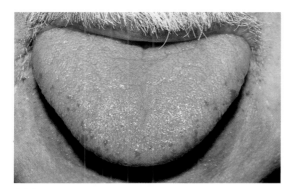

103. A 63-year-old man was admitted with iron-deficiency anaemia.
a. What is the diagnosis?
b. How should it be treated?

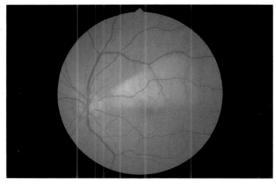

104.
a. What abnormality is shown here?
b. Name two common causes.

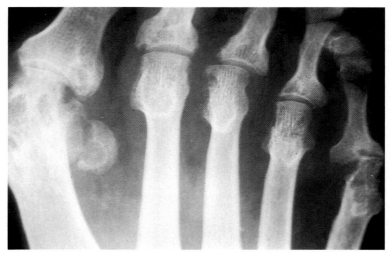

105.
a. Describe the abnormalities shown in this X-ray.
b. What may be the underlying pathological process?

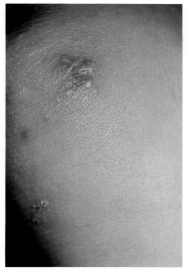

106. A 23-year-old woman developed a generalized rash shown here and a fever a week after a Mediterranean holiday.
a. What is the likely cause?
b. What two other complications can occur?

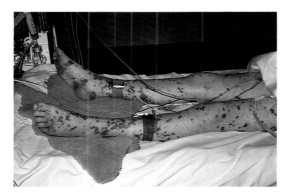

107. This 17-year-old pupil in a boarding school became rapidly very unwell with a febrile illness.
a. What is the cause of the illness?
b. How should it be treated?
c. What other precautions should be taken?

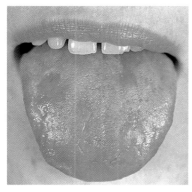

108.
a. What abnormality is shown here?
b. How should it be treated?

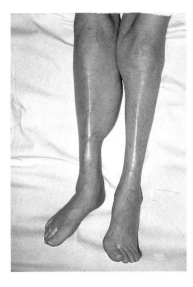

109. This 58-year-old man complained of sudden onset of pain in the right calf.
a. What is the likely diagnosis?
b. What may be the underlying predisposing condition?

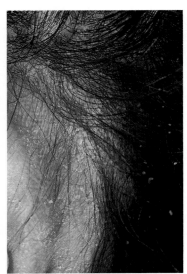

110. This abnormality was found in a 26-year-old man.
a. What is the condition?
b. How should it be treated?

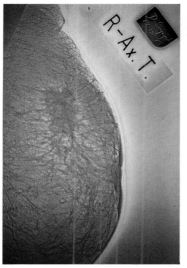

111.
a. What investigation is shown?
b. What abnormality is illustrated?

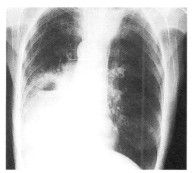

112. A 63-year-old man with a short history of abdominal pain, swinging fever, night sweats and right upper quadrant tenderness had this chest X-ray.
a. What is the likely diagnosis?
b. How should it be treated?

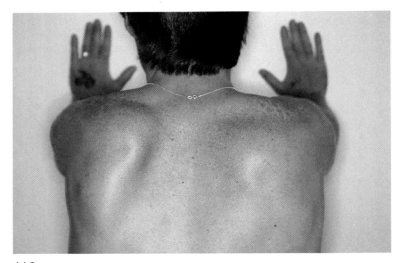

113. **This young man presented with an acute attack of pain in the shoulder.**
a. What abnormality is shown?
b. How may it have been caused?

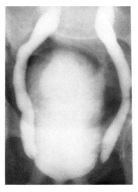 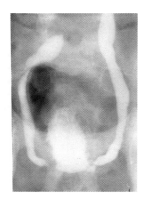

114.
a. What investigation is shown here?
b. What abnormality is shown?

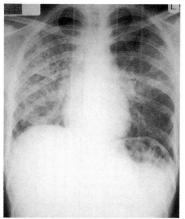

115. This 29-year-old man was admitted with low-grade fever, anorexia, nonproductive cough and progressive dyspnoea.
a. What diagnosis should be considered?
b. What further investigations are appropriate?

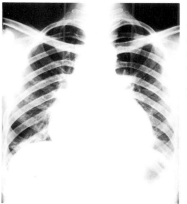

116. A 42-year-old woman, under investigation for malaise, menorrhagia and anaemia, was found to be hypothyroid.
a. What complication does this chest X-ray show?
b. What other sites may be affected similarly?

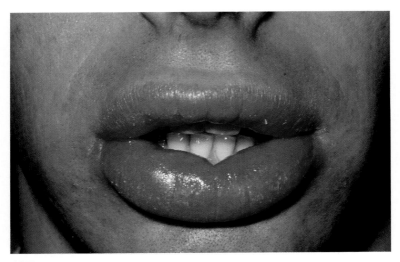

117. This young man feels entirely well, but is being tormented at school because of his appearance which has developed over the previous six months.
a. What underlying disease is present?
b. How should it be treated?

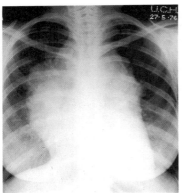

118. This young woman complained of lethargy, sweating and was found to have cervical lymphadenopathy.
a. What does the X-ray show?
b. What is the probable diagnosis?

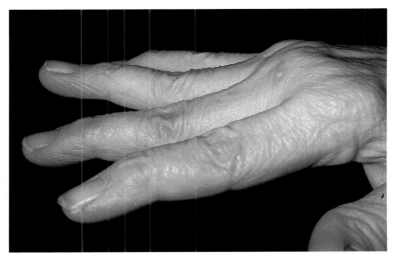

119.
a. What is the name of this abnormality?
b. With what condition is this associated?

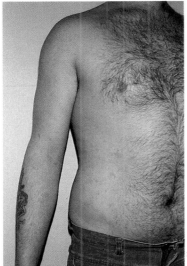

120. **This 32-year-old ex-intravenous drug abuser complained of headaches and arthralgia.**
a. What abnormality is shown?
b. What is its significance?

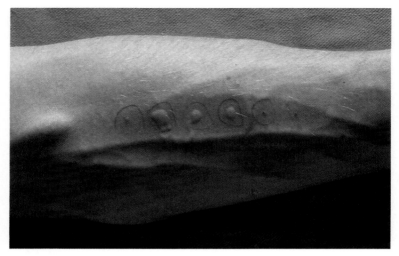

121.
a. What skin test is being undertaken?
b. What does the result shown here indicate?

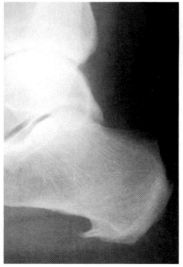

122. A 65-year-old man complained of pain on the sole of his foot on weight bearing.
a. What abnormality is shown?
b. How should it be treated?

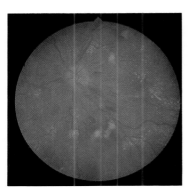

123.
a. What abnormalities are shown in this slide?
b. What is the probable underlying cause?
c. How should it be treated?

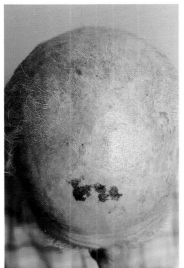

124. This elderly man, who was known to have cirrhosis, developed this lesion on his head and a similar lesion on the dorsal section of his hands.
a. What is this condition?
b. What are the possible underlying causes?

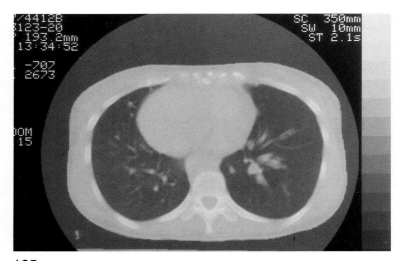

125. **This 30-year-old patient had finger clubbing and a
normal chest radiograph.**
a. What abnormality is shown in this CT scan?
b. What is the cause of the abnormality?

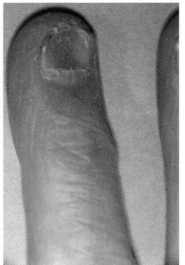

126.
a. What abnormality is shown here?
b. With what is it associated?

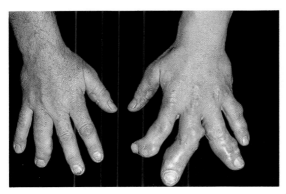

127.
a. What is the cause of this abnormality?
b. What other abnormalities might be found?
c. How is it inherited?

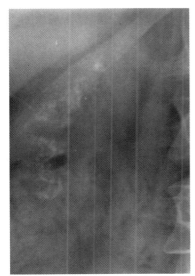

128. **A 15-year-old man with a history of renal colic was found to have a low plasma bicarbonate concentration and hypokalaemia.**

a. What abnormality is shown in the plain abdominal film?
b. What is the likely underlying diagnosis?

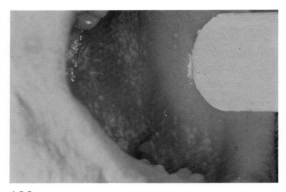

129.
a. What abnormality is shown?
b. How should it be treated?

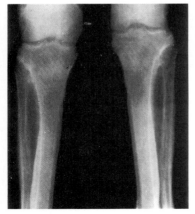

130.
a. What condition is illustrated here?
b. What is the likely underlying diagnosis?

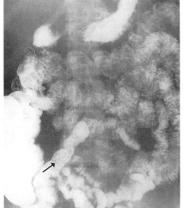

131. A 28-year-old man was investigated for abdominal pain and rectal bleeding.
a. What abnormality is shown on this barium meal?
b. What is the cause of the pain and bleeding?

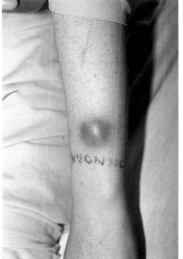

132. This patient had a lung abscess.
a. What three abnormalities are shown?
b. What underlying disorders should be sought?

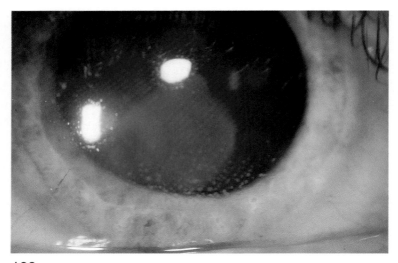

133. **A 48-year-old lady with a five-year history of sarcoidosis complained of painful eyes.**
a. What abnormality is shown?
b. How should it be treated?

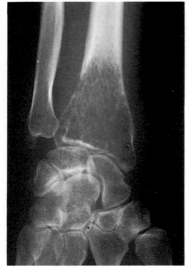

134. This 19-year-old man complained of gradual onset of a painful swollen right wrist.
a. What does the X-ray show?
b. How should it be treated?

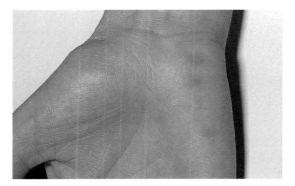

135. A 26-year-old lady presented to Casualty with swinging fever and hypotension.
a. What is the likely cause of the rash?
b. What other investigations are appropriate?

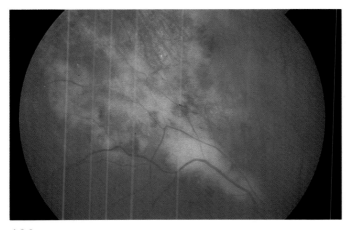

136. A 50-year-old man with severe haemophilia presented with visual loss with no pain, but scotomas were identified on examination.
a. What does fundoscopy show?
b. What may be the underlying cause?

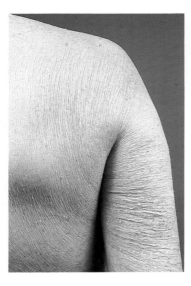

137. This 60-year-old man complained of a recent onset of fatigue, weight loss and skin itching.
a. What is this lesion called?
b. What is the likely associated disease in this case?

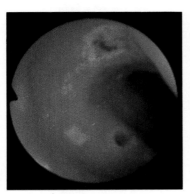

138. This 30-year-old man suffered recurrent relapses of epigastric pain initially responding to ranitidine, but eventually occurring in spite of ranitidine therapy. This was the endoscopic view of his duodenum.
a. What abnormalities are shown?
b. What further investigation is appropriate?

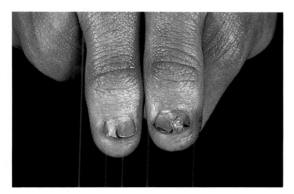

139.
a. What abnormality is shown here?
b. What other skeletal abnormalities may be present?

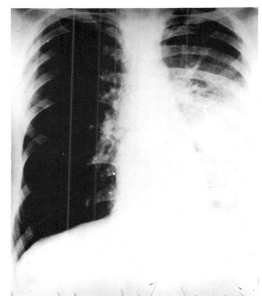

140. A 58-year-old man was admitted to hospital very unwell with malaise, confusion, myalgia and diarrhoea. He had been treated for 2 days with penicillin without response.
a. What important diagnosis should be considered?
b. How should the diagnosis be confirmed?

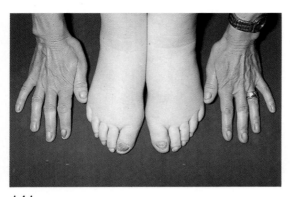

141. This young woman, who had longstanding swelling of her legs, presented with chronic cough.

a. What two abnormalities are shown in this picture?

b. What is this syndrome called?

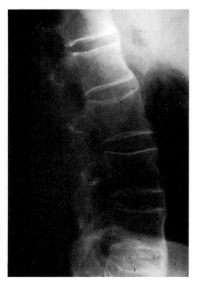

142. A 54-year-old man complained of morning pain and stiffness in his back. Examination showed reduced spinal movement.

a. What abnormality is shown?

b. Name one major extra-articular associated condition.

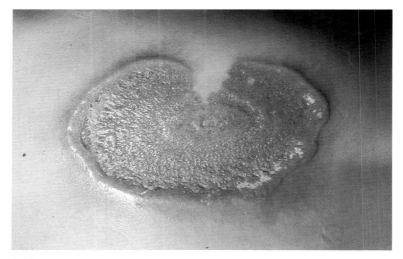

143.
a. What is this lesion?
b. With what condition is it associated?

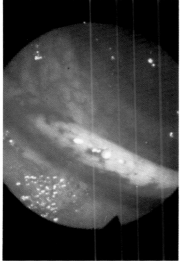

144. This colonoscopic appearance was found in an 82-year-old woman who had been admitted to hospital urgently.
a. What does it show?
b. What was the reason for admission to hospital?

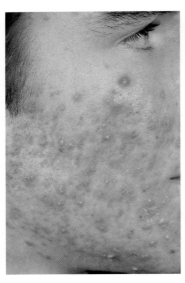

145. This 16-year-old boy complained of a persistent rash on his face and neck.
a. What is the rash?
b. List three factors believed to be important in its aetiology.

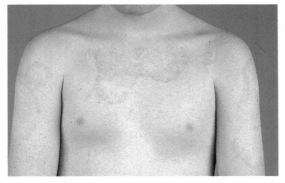

146.
a. What abnormality is shown?
b. How may it be treated?

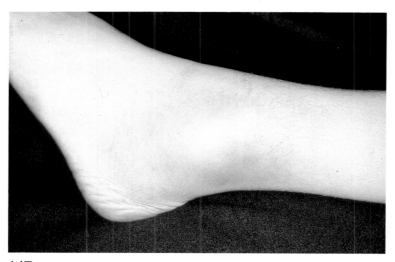

147. A 13-year-old boy presented to the Accident &
Emergency Department with pain in the left ankle associated
with pyrexia.
a. What is the likely cause of the pain?
b. What investigations are indicated?

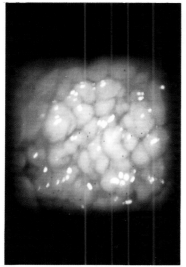

148. A 33-year-old man with
chronic epigastric pain
underwent an upper GI
endoscopy.
a. What is the probable diagnosis?
b. How should the diagnosis be
confirmed?

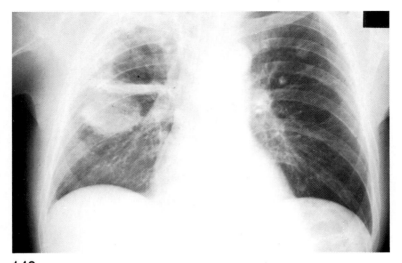

149. This 26-year-old man presented with fever and rigors.
a. What is the lesion shown?
b. Give two underlying causes.

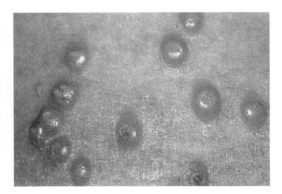

150. This otherwise well man presented with these painless, but extensive lesions on his face.
a. What are the lesions shown in this figure?
b. What underlying cause may predispose to this condition?

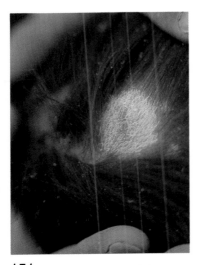

151. This 14-year-old boy complained of patchy alopecia.
a. What investigation is being shown here?
b. What abnormality is present?

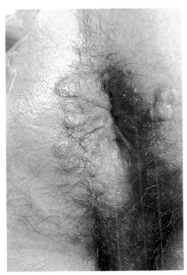

152.
a. What are the lesions shown?
b. With what condition is this associated?
c. How should this be treated?

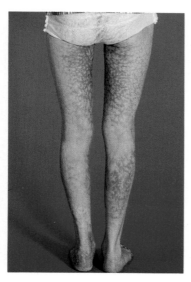

153.
a. What physical sign is illustrated here?
b. What is its significance?

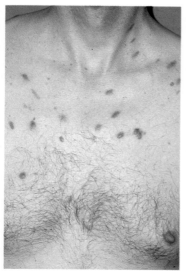

154. This patient has moderately severe haemophilia.
a. What is this lesion?
b. With what condition is it associated?
c. What is its significance?

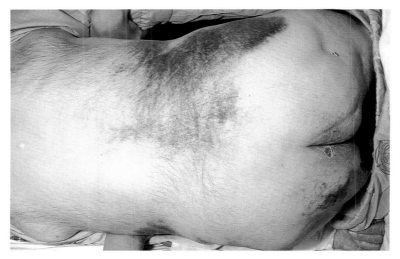

155.
a. What is the cause of this physical sign?
b. Name one condition which may cause this sign.

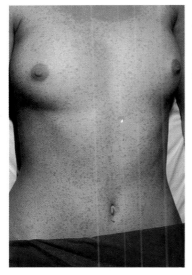

156. This woman suffered an upper respiratory infection with conjunctivitis and then developed this rash.
a. What is the diagnosis?
b. What other abnormality is often found?

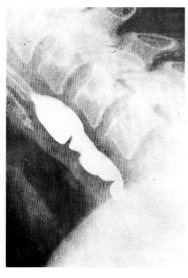

157. This patient presented with dysphagia.
a. What abnormality is shown?
b. What may be the underlying condition?

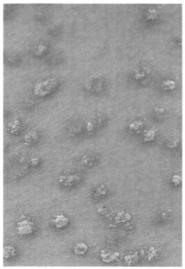

158.
a. What variant of a common skin disorder does this show?
b. What preceding precipitating illness may have occurred?

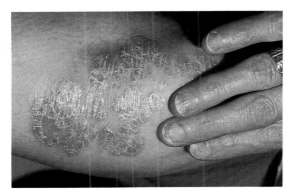

159.
a. What two abnormalities are shown in the picture?
b. Name two other causes of the appearance in the fingers.

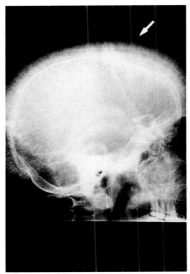

160. This 17-year-old man from the Middle East complained of left upper quadrant abdominal pain.
a. What does the X-ray show?
b. What is the underlying diagnosis?

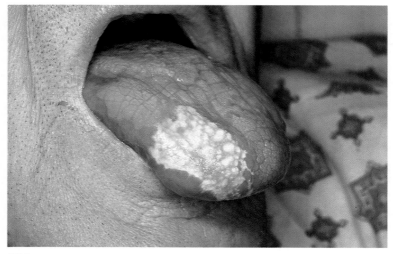

161.
a. What is the lesion shown here?
b. With what conditions may it be associated?

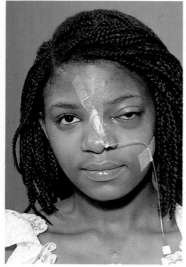

162. **This 19-year-old girl complained of persistent headache following a cold.**
a. What abnormality is shown?
b. How should it be treated?

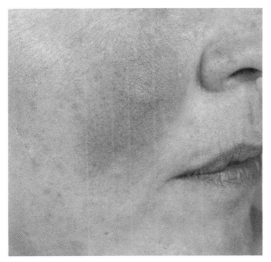

163.
a. What abnormality is shown?
b. With what condition is this associated?
c. What treatment may be used?

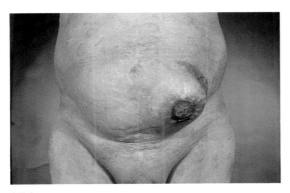

164. This patient had an ileostomy after colectomy for ulcerative colitis.
a. What is unusual about the stoma?
b. How has this led to peripheral skin atrophy?

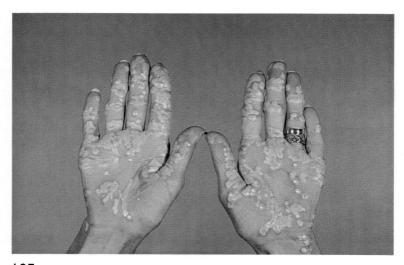

165. This 58-year-old alcoholic lady was found also to have primary biliary cirrhosis. She complained of painful paraesthesia of her hands.
a. What is the likely diagnosis?
b. How should it be treated?

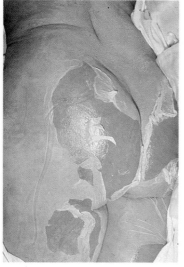

166.
a. What is the abnormality shown?
b. What predisposing disorder may be present?

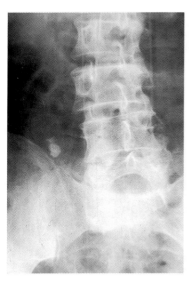

167. This is a plain X-ray of a patient presenting with abdominal pain.
a. What abnormality is shown?
b. What investigations should be undertaken?

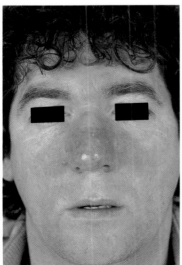

168.
a. What is the condition shown here?
b. How should it be treated?

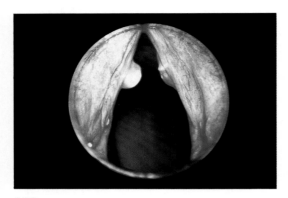

169. **A 42-year-old auctioneer complained of hoarseness.**
a. What abnormality is shown?
b. How should it be treated?

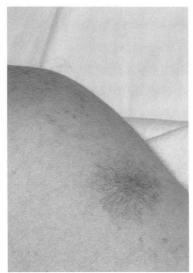

170.
a. What physical sign is shown here?
b. What is its significance?

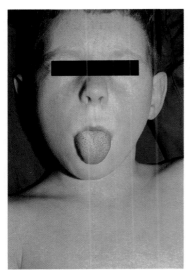

171.
a. What abnormality is shown in this figure?
b. With what condition is it associated?

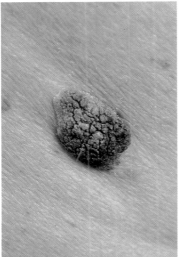

172. A middle-aged woman presented because this asymptomatic lesion had slowly increased in size over several months.
a. What is the lesion?
b. How should it be treated?

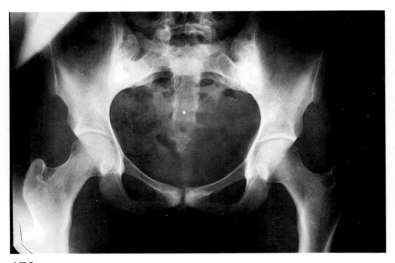

173. **A 36-year-old man, who had recently been troubled with eye problems, complained of back pain.**
a. What is the underlying diagnosis?
b. What investigation is indicated?

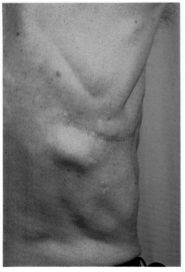

174. **This retired shipyard worker complained of increasing breathlessness.**
a. List the abnormalities shown.
b. With what condition may this be associated?

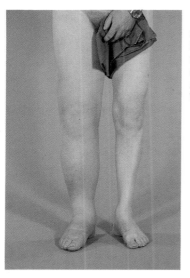

175. **A 41-year-old man was found during a routine insurance medical examination to show the following clinical sign.**
a. What is the likely diagnosis?
b. What is the cause?

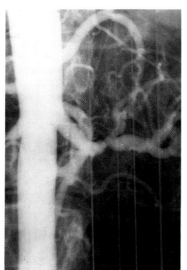

176. **This renal angiogram was obtained in a 42-year-old man with hypertension.**
a. What abnormality is shown?
b. What percentage of patients with hypertension have this as an underlying cause?

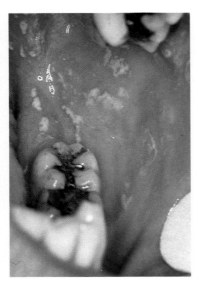

177.
a. What is the abnormality?
b. List three possible underlying causes.

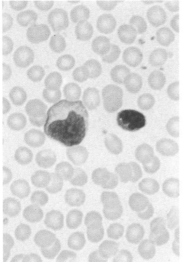

178.
A 19-year-old woman was seen on account of an acute onset of malaise, sore throat and fever. The spleen tip was palpable and the liver function tests were abnormal. A peripheral blood film was taken and is illustrated.
a. What abnormality is shown?
b. What is the underlying diagnosis?

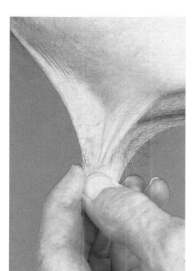

179.
a. What underlying disorder is present here?
b. List three other features that should be looked for.

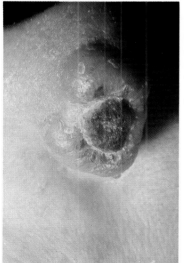

180. A 71-year-old lady was referred to the Dermatology Clinic with this lesion on the side of her neck.
a. What is the abnormality?
b. How should it be treated?

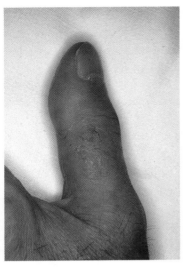

181. A 52-year-old man being treated for rheumatoid arthritis complained of this scaly, itchy rash.
a. What is the likely cause?
b. How should it be treated?

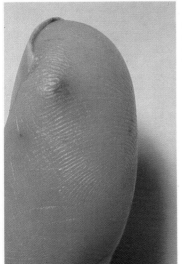

182. A 37-year-old man was admitted with weight loss, sweats and arthralgia.
a. What physical sign is shown?
b. What is the underlying pathology?

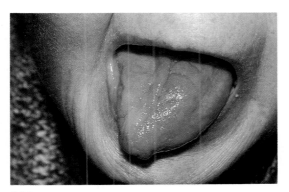

183.
a. What abnormality is shown?
b. What is the underlying cause?

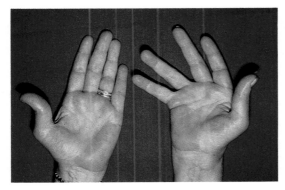

184.
a. What abnormalities are illustrated here?
b. What condition requires exclusion?

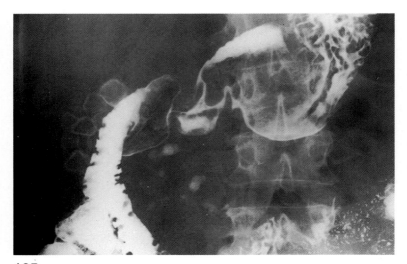

185. A 43-year-old man with a four-year history of episodic severe abdominal pain was admitted for further investigation.
a. What two extraintestinal abnormalities are shown in this X-ray?
b. What two further investigations are appropriate?

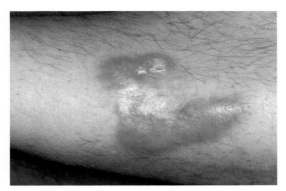

186. A middle-aged woman presented with this slowly enlarging lesion.
a. What part of the body is usually affected?
b. What underlying condition did she have?

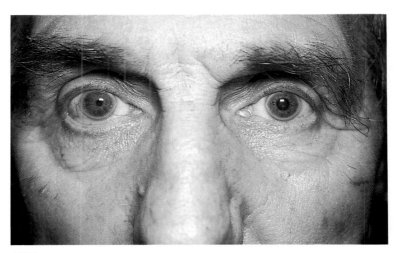

187. A 67-year-old retired coal miner complained of loss of energy. His general practitioner noted the abnormality shown and finger clubbing.
a. What physical sign is shown?
b. What underlying pathology should be sought?

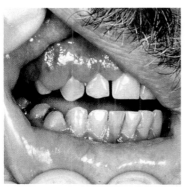

188. This 32-year-old man complained of fatigue, and examination showed pallor and diffuse petechiae
a. What does this figure show?
b. What is the likely underlying cause?
c. What single investigation would confirm the diagnosis?

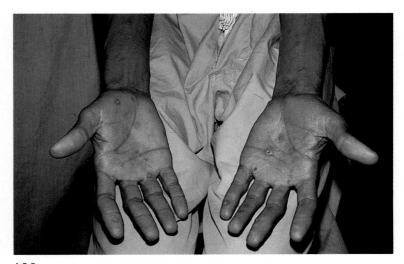

189. A 42-year-old merchant seaman saw his general practitioner complaining of a skin rash and of feeling nonspecifically unwell with mild weight loss.
a. What is the likely cause of the rash?
b. How should this be confirmed?

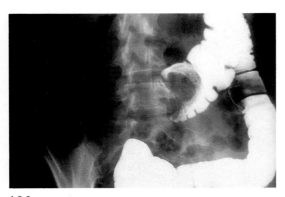

190. A 23-year-old man was admitted with recurrent attacks of colicky abdominal pain.
a. What does the X-ray show?
b. How should it be treated?

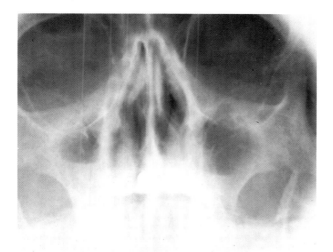

191.

a. What abnormality is shown in this X-ray?
b. How should it be treated?

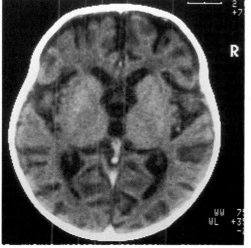

192. This is the CT scan of a 27-year-old man complaining of mild headache and progressive confusion.

a. What abnormality is shown?
b. What underlying diagnosis should be considered?

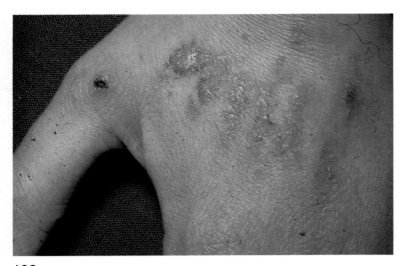

193. **A 17-year-old girl was admitted for the third time to her local hospital with self poisoning. This abnormality was detected on the back of her hand.**
a. What is the diagnosis?
b. What two therapeutic interventions should be instituted?

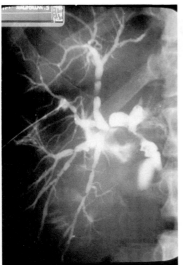

194. **This 62-year-old man was referred by his general practitioner with jaundice, low-grade fever and diarrhoea.**
a. What investigation is illustrated?
b. What is the probable diagnosis?

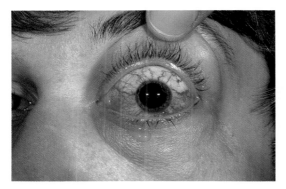

195.
a. What is the abnormality shown?
b. What may be the underlying cause?

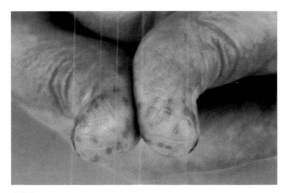

196. This 21-year-old man was admitted to hospital with melaena.
a. What abnormality is shown here?
b. Name one other site showing this change.
c. What was the source of the bleeding?

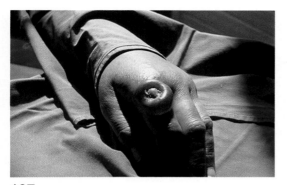

197. A 28-year-old shepherdess
presented to her general
practitioner with this irritating
but pain-free nodule.
a. What is the likely diagnosis?
b. How should it be treated?

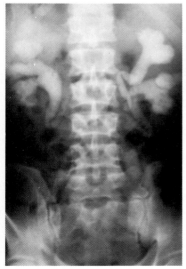

198. This intravenous urogram
was obtained from an
asymptomatic patient known to
have chronic renal failure.
a. What abnormality is shown?
b. Suggest two possible causes?

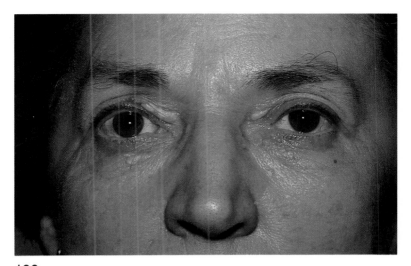

199. A 53-year-old lady with a long history of pruritis had this appearance.
a. What abnormality is present?
b. What is the likely underlying diagnosis?

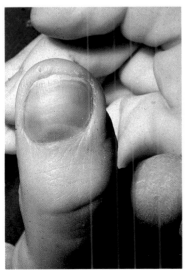

200. A 46-year-old man complained of an exquisitely tender area at the tip of his thumb which was very sensitive to heat and cold. There was no history of trauma.
a. What is the underlying diagnosis?
b. How should it be treated?

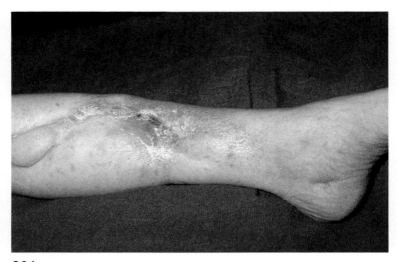

201.
A 40-year-old man injured his leg in a road traffic accident 12 years ago. He has been feeling increasingly fatigued over a year and investigation shows heavy proteinuria.
a. What is illustrated in this figure?
b. What complication has arisen?

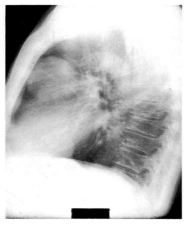

202.
This 23-year-old lady complained of tiredness and weakness.
a. What abnormality does the X-ray show?
b. How does this explain her symptoms?

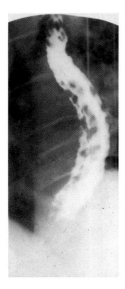

203. This 46-year-old woman presented to Accident & Emergency with melaena.
a. What abnormality is shown in this barium swallow?
b. How should this patient be managed?

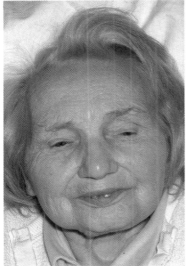

204. This elderly lady developed pneumonia and became hypotensive and hypothermic.
a. What features were illustrated?
b. What may be the underlying cause?

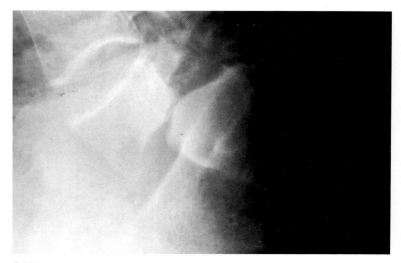

205. This 31-year-old man complained of a long history of lower back pain.
a. What is the diagnosis?
b. How may it be treated?

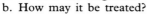

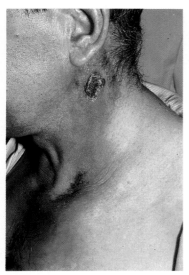

206. A 41-year-old professional gardener complained of fever and inguinal lymphadenopathy.
a. What abnormality is illustrated?
b. What is the underlying diagnosis?

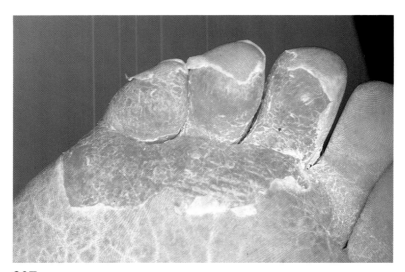

207. This 26-year-old man complained to his general practitioner about itchy toes.
a. What is the underlying cause of this abnormality?
b. How should it be treated?

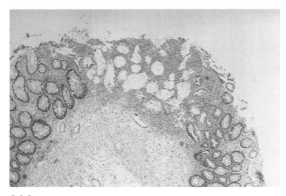

208. A 54-year-old lady who was in an intensive care unit following cardiac surgery complained of severe watery diarrhoea on the 10th postoperative day. A rectal biopsy was taken.
a. What is the diagnosis?
b. How should it be treated?

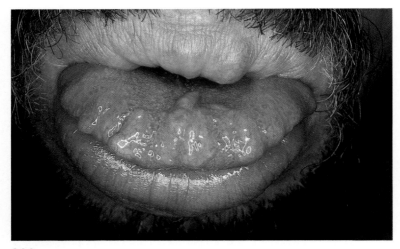

209. **This patient was found to have a medullary thyroid carcinoma.**
a. What abnormality of the tongue is shown?
b. Name two associated conditions?

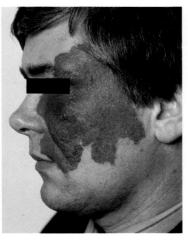

210.
a. What is the abnormality shown?
b. What syndrome may be associated?
c. What are the syndrome's other features?

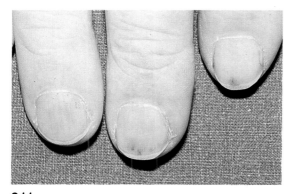

211. **This lady presented with fever, weight loss, feeling generally unwell, and renal failure.**
a. What abnormality is shown in the figure?
b. What is the cause of the patient's illness?
c. What is the cause of the renal failure?

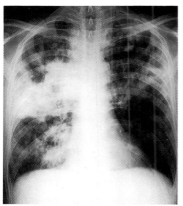

212. **This patient has had prolonged corticosteroid treatment for bronchial asthma.**
a. What complication has occurred?
b. What may be the underlying problem?

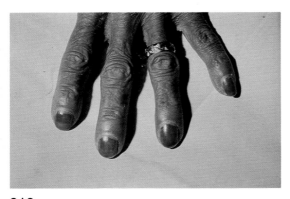

213. **A 53-year-old lady complained of tiredness and severe persistent itching.**
a. What two abnormalities are shown?
b. What is the likely underlying disease?

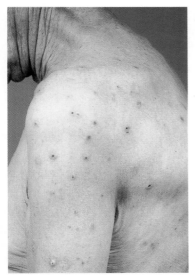

214. **This rash was observed in a 61-year-old homeless man.**
a. What is the probable underlying cause?
b. How should it be treated?

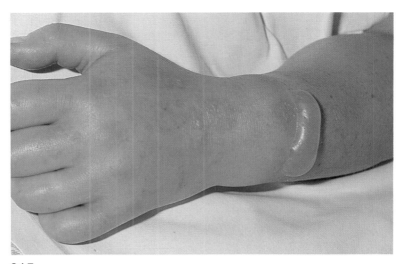

215. A 19-year-old lady was found collapsed at home.
a. What abnormality is shown?
b. What is the likely diagnosis?

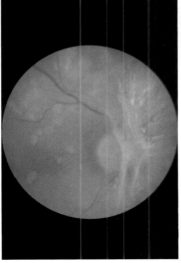

216. A 26-year-old insulin-dependent diabetic with poor diabetic control was seen for his annual appointment.
a. What abnormality is shown?
b. What complications may arise?

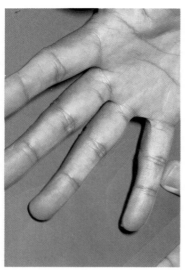

217. **This patient complained of tiredness, anorexia and weight loss and had a BP of 95/50.**
a. What was the cause of his illness?
b. Name three other sites which may show this physical sign.

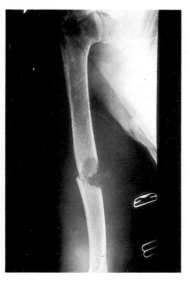

218.
a. What abnormalities are shown in this X-ray?
b. What investigations should be undertaken?

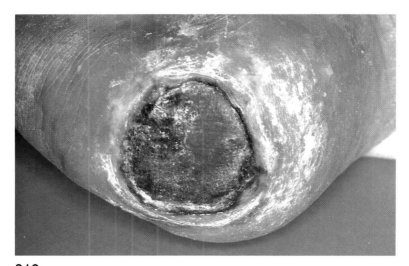

219. This shows a persistent ulcer on the heel of a foot of a 62-year-old man.
a. What is the likely underlying disorder?
b. What factors contribute to the ulcer formation?

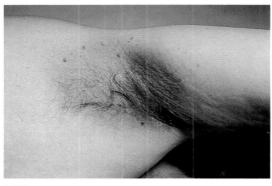

220.
a. What physical sign is shown here?
b. What is its significance?

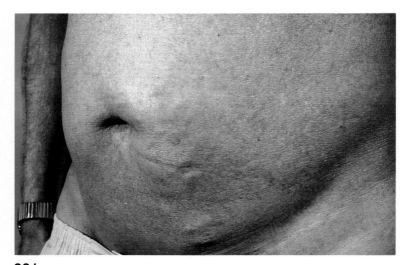

221. A 55-year-old man presented to the Accident & Emergency Department with a major haematemesis.
a. What physical sign is illustrated in this slide?
b. What is the probable underlying cause?
c. How should the bleeding be treated?

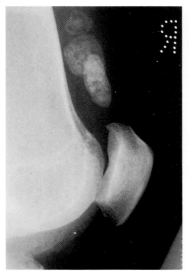

222. This 46-year-old man complained of a swollen right knee which locked unpredictably.
a. What is the diagnosis?
b. How should it be treated?

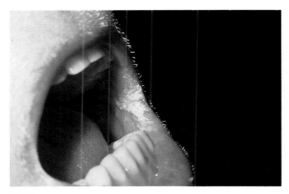

223.
a. What abnormality of the lips is shown?
b. What is its significance?

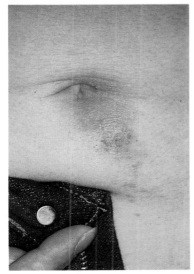

224. This 16-year-old girl complained of an itchy patch below her umbilicus.
a. Name the lesion.
b. What is the likely cause?

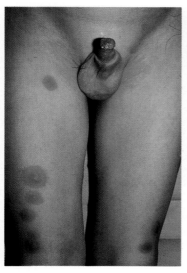

225.
a. What abnormalities are shown in this figure?
b. List three possible causes.

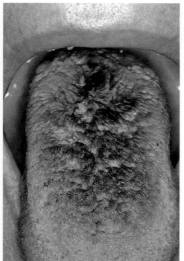

226.
a. What abnormality is illustrated?
b. How should it be treated?

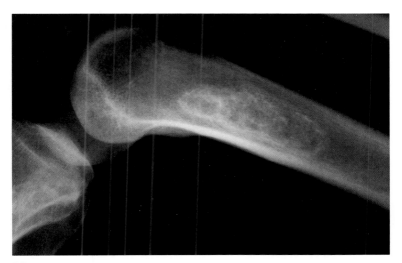

227. A 47-year-old man with a long history of alcohol abuse and who had had corticosteroid treatment for a number of years for asthma was found to have the following abnormality.
a. What is the cause of the abnormality?
b. What symptoms may be present?

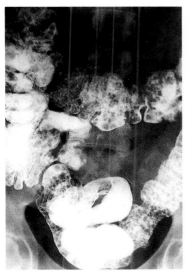

228. A 26-year-old man presented with intermittent rectal bleeding. His father had died of colon cancer aged 46 years.
a. What does this barium enema show?
b. What is the underlying diagnosis?

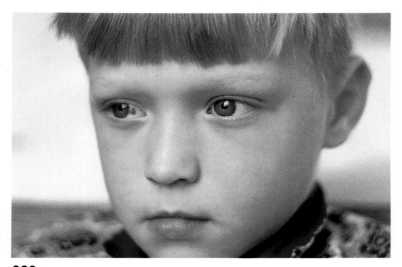

229. This six-year-old boy was taken to his general practitioner by his mother who said his cough had been getting worse over the preceding week.

a. What physical sign is present?
b. What underlying diagnosis should be considered?

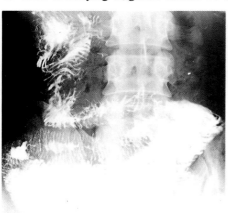

230. A 65-year-old lady complained of longstanding abdominal discomfort and dysphagia. She was found to have malabsorption.

a. What abnormality is illustrated?
b. What is the most likely underlying diagnosis?

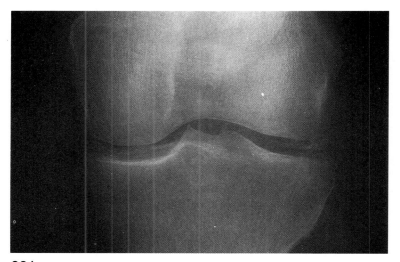

231. **A 61-year-old man complained of pain and swelling in his right knee.**
a. What abnormality is shown?
b. What is the probable underlying diagnosis?

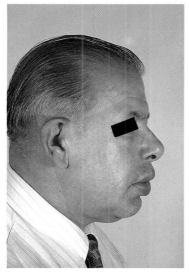

232. **This 58-year-old man complained of recurrent episodes of facial swelling.**
a. What is the diagnosis?
b. How should severe acute attacks be treated?
c. What is the underlying biochemical abnormality?

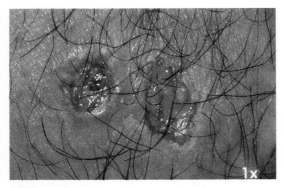

233. **A 35-year-old man complained to his GP of these lesions on his scrotum.**
a. What abnormality is shown?
b. What is the likely underlying diagnosis?

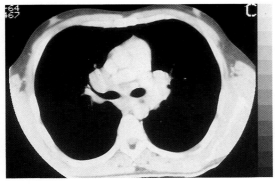

234.
a. What abnormality is shown on the CT scan?
b. What are the two most important causes?

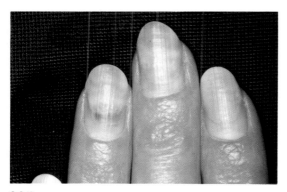

235.
a. What abnormality is shown?
b. List three underlying causes.

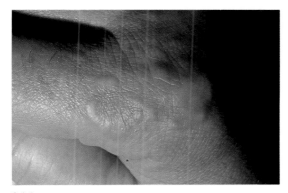

236. This is the hand of a patient with diabetes mellitus.
a. What abnormality is shown?
b. What is it due to?

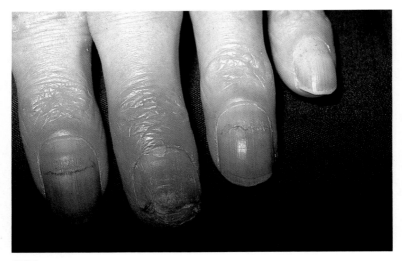

237.
a. What is the name of the abnormality here?
b. What is the underlying cause?

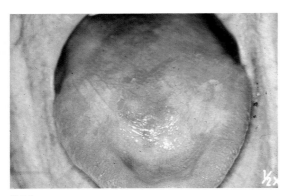

238. This 74-year-old woman complained of tiredness and she then consulted her doctor because of difficulty in walking.
a. What abnormality is shown?
b. What is the likely cause?

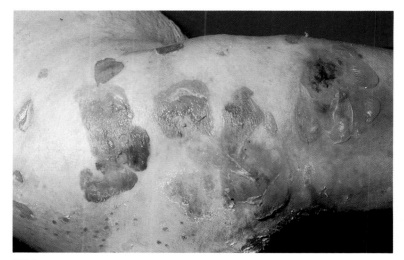

239.
a. What is the abnormality shown?
b. What diagnostic sign can be used to confirm the diagnosis?

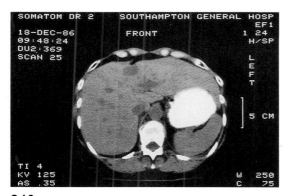

240. A 68-year-old man presented with a recent history of weight loss. His liver was palpable and a CT scan was done.
a. What is the likely diagnosis?
b. What two further tests would you do?

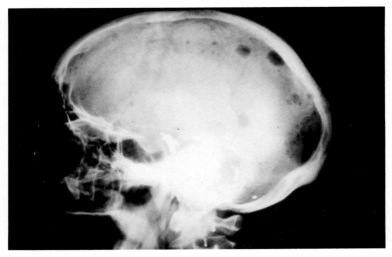

241.
a. What abnormality is illustrated in this radiograph?
b. What is the likely underlying diagnosis?
c. How should this be confirmed?

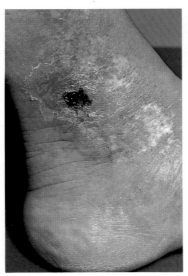

242. This 74-year-old lady complained of recurrent sores on the medial aspect of her lower leg.
a. What is the abnormality shown?
b. What is the probable underlying cause?

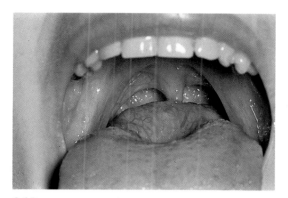

243. A 23-year-old woman complained of progressive dysphagia.
a. What abnormality is illustrated?
b. What other investigation is necessary before treatment?

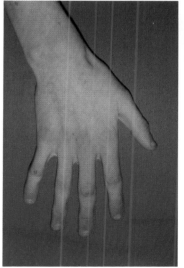

244. This tall patient has aortic incompetence.
a. What abnormality is shown in this photograph?
b. What is the underlying diagnosis?

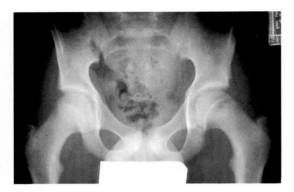

245. This 15-year-old boy who was a keen footballer complained of pain in the left hip.
a. What does the X-ray show?
b. What complication may arise?

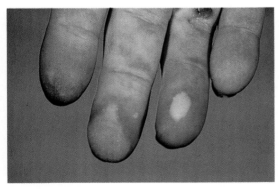

246.
a. Describe the abnormality shown.
b. How should it be treated?

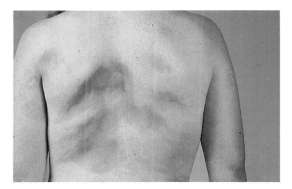

247. This young woman had noticed these lesions gradually worsening over many months.
a. What is the abnormality?
b. What underlying disease causes this lesion?

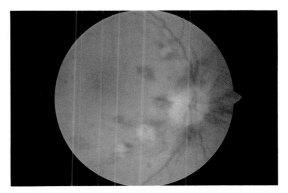

248. This is the fundoscopic appearance of an elderly patient admitted with severe anaemia.
a. What abnormality is shown?
b. What is the likely diagnosis?

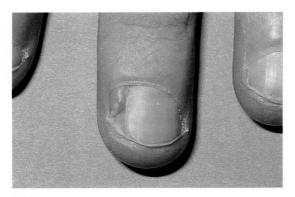

249.
a. What abnormality is shown?
b. What is the underlying disorder?

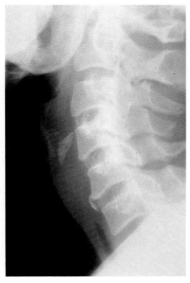

250. A 33-year-old man complained of pain on swallowing which he localized to the neck.
a. What abnormality is shown?
b. Name three complications of this occurrence.

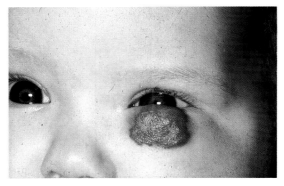

251.
a. What abnormality is shown here?
b. How should it be treated?

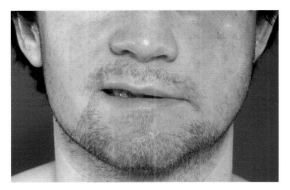

252. This 26-year-old, past intravenous drug abuser complained of general ill health.
a. What abnormality is shown here?
b. What underlying condition should be considered?

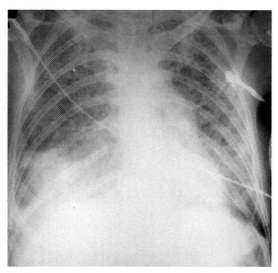

253. **This patient was admitted to hospital with acute pancreatitis 48 hours before this radiograph was taken.**
a. What abnormality is shown?
b. What did his arterial blood P_{O_2}, P_{CO_2} and pH show?

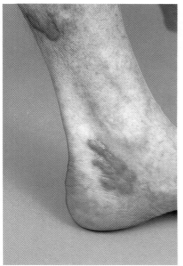

254. **This 46-year-old man who has recently been made redundant complained of this itchy eruption on his ankle.**
a. What is this abnormality?
b. How should it be treated?

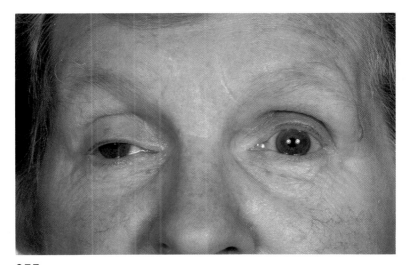

255. This abnormality resolved fully after two months of medical therapy.
a. What abnormality is shown?
b. What underlying condition was the cause?

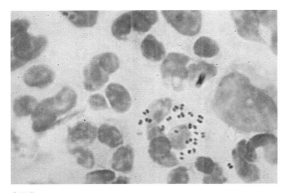

256. This is a Gram stain of a urethral smear on a 23-year-old man.
a. What is the diagnosis?
b. How should it be confirmed?

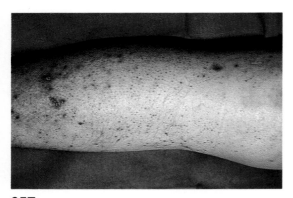

257. An elderly widower was admitted to Accident & Emergency.
a. What abnormality is shown? What is the characteristic site of these lesions?
b. How should it be treated? Name two other manifestations of this disease.

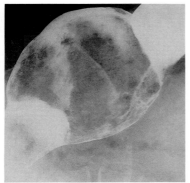

258. This 17-year-old man had complained of constipation since childhood.
a. What does this investigation show?
b. What is the probable underlying cause?

Answers

1.
  a. This is a maculopapular eruption typical of a drug reaction.
  b. Drugs likely to have caused this include ampicillin, particularly in those with glandular fever, other antibiotics and phenothiazines.

2.
  a. Enamel hypoplasia.
  b. This is associated with tuberous sclerosis, which may be the underlying cause of the epilepsy.

3.
  a. Peroneal muscular atrophy or Charcot–Marie–Tooth disease.
  b. Autosomal dominant trait.

4.
  a. Crops of papules, vesicles and pustules.
  b. Chickenpox.

5.
  a. Trichomonal vaginitis.
  b. Metronidazole.

6.
  a. Digital gangrene.
  b. Vasculitis as in rheumatoid disease, Raynaud's disease, cold injury, cryoglobulinaemia.

7.
  a. Severe leg ulcers with associated skin pigmentation and arthritis of the toes.
  b. Felty's syndrome.

8.
  a. A typical herpetic lesion on the neck.
  b. Herpes simplex virus (type I usually) encephalitis.
  c. Patients should be treated with acyclovir at the first clinical suspicion and with steroids to control raised intracranial pressure. Anticonvulsants may be necessary in some patients. Despite this treatment mortality remains high and neurological sequelae are common.

9.
  a. Bilateral thenar wasting.
  b. Bilateral carpal tunnel syndrome.

10.
  a. Acromegaly.
  b. Enlarged feet, prognathia, coarsening of features, enlarged tongue, hypertension, cardiac failure.

11.
  a. Ochronotic pigment in sclerae.
  b. Alkaptonuria.

12.
a. Superior vena caval obstruction.
b. Radiotherapy is often a valuable palliatitive treatment, reducing obstruction.

13.
a. Acne, hirsutism and seborrhoea indicate benign androgen excess or the Stein-Leventhal syndrome. This is a common disorder affecting around 1% of the female population with increased ovarian androgen production resulting in hirsutism.
b. The differential diagnoses includes congenital adrenal hyperplasia, ovarian tumours e.g. hilus cell tumour and arrhenoblastoma and virilising adrenal tumours.

14.
a. A fluid level in a dilated oesophagus and an absent gastric bubble.
b. Achalasia can be treated by pneumatic dilatation or by surgery (Heller's operation).

15.
a. Acanthocytosis or Burr cells.
b. This may be inherited as an autosomal recessive abnormality associated with retinitis pigmentosa, neurological deficits and a beta-lipoproteinaemia. It may also occur in chronic renal failure, cirrhosis, microangiopathic haemolytic anaemia, and as an artifact with blood stored in EDTA.

16.
a. An osteochondroma of the proximal tibia.
b. This is the commonest benign bone tumour often found near the knee. If troublesome the lesion can be removed surgically.

17.
a. Osteopetrosis.
b. Bone fractures starting in childhood are common.

18.
a. Disc pallor due to optic atrophy.
b. a) Demyelinating disease e.g. MS, b) optic neuritis, c) ischaemic optic neuropathy, d) secondary optic atrophy related to unrelieved papilloedema.

19.
a. Eruptive xanthomatosis.
b. These usually resolve in a month or two of treating the hyperglycaemia.

20.
a. Wegener's granulomatosis.
b. Biopsy of the nasal mucosa or lung, anti-neutrophil cytoplasmic antibodies.

21.
a. Larva migrans.
b. The most commonly involved areas are the skin of the feet, hands or buttocks.

c. The most likely cause is a reaction to various worms, e.g. *Angylostoma braziliense* or *Strongyloides stercoralis*, which penetrate the skin and then migrate producing itchy, raised, red, serpentine lines.

22.
a. This figure illustrates swelling of the elbow joint due to acute arthritis with erythema nodosum on the forearm.
b. The most likely diagnosis particularly with regard to the hypercalcaemia is sarcoidosis. Further investigations should include chest X-ray which will show hilar lymphadenopathy in 75% of patients, rheumatoid factor which may be positive in 10% and a biopsy of synovium or other affected tissues which will show granulomata and inflammatory changes.

23.
a. Anginose pharyngitis with wash-leather exudate, typical of infectious mononucleosis.
b. Cervical lymphadenopathy and palatal petechiae are common.

24.
a. A paravertebral abscess seen behind the heart shadow.
b. Investigations should include a Mantoux test and aspiration of the abscess and culture of material obtained. The blood count should be checked and the ESR is usually high during active infection.

25.
a. Histology of melanosis coli showing brown pigment.
b. Laxative abuse.

26.
a. Acrosclerosis of the skin which becomes hard and tightly bound down. The fingers become tapered and shiny with loss of finger pulps (sclerodactyly).
b. This is a classical feature of progressive systemic sclerosis which is a multisystem disease of unknown cause, thought to be autoimmune.

27.
a. Weakness and wasting of the muscles around the shoulders.
b. Fascioscapulohumeral dystrophy.

28.
a. Pathological cupping of the optic disc.
b. Examination of visual fields may identify peripheral field loss in patients with glaucoma leading to tunnel vision.

29.
a. Purpura.
b. Drug therapy. Salazopyrin occasionally causes mild Heinz-body anaemia and neutropenia, and rarely thrombocytopenia or agranulocytosis.

30.
a. The burrow of the mite of scabies can be seen as can secondary lesions due to scratching.
b. Infection with *Sarcoptes scabiei hominis*.

31.
a. Periileostomy varices.
b. Immediate treatment is by local pressure and ligation. Long term treatment by portasystemic shunt surgery or transjugular intrahepatic portasystemic shunt (TIPSS) should be considered in patients with adequate hepatic function as hepatic encephalopathy is rare after colectomy.

32.
a. This plain abdominal film shows a toxic megacolon with finger printing.
b. Ischaemic colitis.

33.
a. Positive Froment's sign in the left hand.
b. This is diagnostic of an ulnar nerve lesion. The sign is caused by the flexor pollicis longus (innervated by the median nerve) which comes into action when the patient attempts to grip a flat object between the thumb and the hand, and causes flexion at the interphalangeal joint.

34.
a. Myelinated nerve fibres.
b. Papilloedema.
c. None.

35.
a. Right adrenal calcification.
b. Right adrenal carcinoma.

36.
a. Hypertrophy of the distal cutaneous branch of the sural nerve in the lateral border of the foot.
b. Hypertrophy of the cutaneous nerves is found in chronic demyelinating neuropathies and in leprosy (Hansen's disease).

37.
a. Wasting of the small muscles of the hand.
b. Motor neurone disease.

38.
a. Multiple cysts in both kidneys.
b. Intracranial vascular malformations may be present.

39.
a. Short fourth metacarpal (brachydactyly).
b. Pseudohypoparathyroidism.

40.
a. A middle-ear effusion.
b. It is commonly associated with obstruction of the eustachian tube, due either to acute upper respiratory tract infections or chronically in children with adenoid hypertrophy. In adults, middle-ear effusions may be due to eustachian tube obstruction by nasopharyngeal tumours.

41.
a. Perianal abscesses and sinuses.
b. Crohn's disease.

42.
a. Kayser–Fleischer rings.
b. Urinary copper which is increased, and plasma caeruloplasmin which is reduced.

43.
a. Discoid eczema.
b. Aetiological factors include: stress, overwashing, and conditions of low humidity as with air conditioning and central heating.

44.
a. Fracture of the scaphoid bone.
b. If a fracture of the scaphoid is suspected but not confirmed on X-ray, the wrist should still be placed in plaster and a further examination carried out in 10 days. Fractures of the scaphoid usually will unite after splintage for 6 weeks, but occasionally bone grafting may be necessary for delayed union.

45.
a. A dorsoradial wrist ganglion.
b. About one-half of ganglia disappear spontaneously. Aspiration or excision is indicated if the ganglion is symptomatic or large, but recurrence is not uncommon.

46.
a. Tibial exostosis.
b. Gardner's syndrome. A variant of familial adenomatous polyposis.

47.
a. Acute peritonsillar abscess (quinsy).
b. Once an abscess has formed, incision and drainage and intravenous benzylpenicillin are necessary.

48.
a. Tonic (Holmes-Adie) pupil syndrome.
b. This is an entirely benign condition which is most common in young women. It is associated with diminished deep tendon reflexes.

49.
a. Leukonychia.
b. It is associated with hypoalbuminaemia as may occur in liver disease and nephrotic syndrome. It is also seen in chronic inorganic arsenic poisoning.

50.
a. Osteoarthrosis with formation of osteophytes, bone cysts, sclerosis and joint space loss and narrowing.
b. Treatment for chronic arthritis should include analgesics, antiinflammatory drugs, physiotherapy and advice regarding aids and appliances. Many patients, however, will require a hip prosthesis to alleviate pain and promote mobility.

51.
a. Bilateral calf hypertrophy.
b. Duchenne muscular dystrophy.

52.
a. An enlarged tongue.
b. Amyloidosis.
c. Biopsy with histological confirmation showing eosinophilic hyaline material with a fibrillar structure on ultramicroscopy.

53.
a. Facial flushing.
b. Marked hepatomegaly.
c. 24-hour urine 5HIAA to confirm the diagnosis of carcinoid syndrome.

54.
a. Retinitis pigmentosa.
b. It may be associated with Friedreich's ataxia, Laurence-Moon-Biedl syndrome or Refsum's syndrome.

55.
a. Pulmonary haemosiderosis.

56.
a. Myotonic dystrophy.
b. Typical features are ptosis, weakness and wasting of muscles of the face, distal limbs and sternomastoids. Associated conditions are cardiac arrhythmias, oesophageal atresia, constipation, glucose intolerance, testicular atrophy and frontal baldness.

57.
a. Gynaecomastia.
b. Ectopic gonadotrophin associated with a bronchial carcinoma.
c. Serum gonadotrophin levels.

58.
a. This radiograph shows multiple discrete osteoblastic metastases throughout the pelvis.
b. A number of tumours may produce osteosclerotic lesions on X-ray but prostatic carcinoma is the commonest and the most likely in this case. Investigations should include needle aspiration of the prostate for histology and the serum acid phosphatase level.

59.
a. Late Volkmann's ischaemic contracture.
b. Ischaemia of the muscles in the forearm occurs because of interruption to the arterial supply or venous drainage; in this case, and most commonly, after a supracondylar fracture of the humerus in children.

60.
a. Papilloedema.
b. Raised intracranial pressure due most commonly to intracranial tumours or hydrocephalus, and accelerated hypertension.

61.
a. A pharyngeal pouch.
b. Complications include dysphagia and pneumonia secondary to pulmonary aspiration.

62.
a. Pectus excavatum.
b. This may be cosmetically distressing, but is of little functional significance.

63.
  a. A collarstud abscess.
  b. Tuberculosis, the underlying cause, should be confirmed by Mantoux test and identifying the organism from material from the abscess or other infected material such as sputum.

64.
  a. There is a large multiloculated frontal lobe abscess showing ring enhancement and midline shift.
  b. Cerebral abscesses may result from direct spread of infection from the paranasal sinuses, teeth, middle ear or mastoid region, or may be blood borne from lung disease e.g. bronchiectasis or tuberculosis or from heart disease e.g. bacterial endocarditis. The most commonly incriminated organisms are streptococci, staphylococci and anaerobes.

65.
  a. Dark-ground microscopy showing *Treponema pallidum*.
  b. Serological tests such as the TPHA and FTA-Abs.

66.
  a. Nail dystrophy.
  b. Cronkhite-Canada syndrome.

67.
  a. Left subdural haemorrhage with displacement of the left hemisphere across the midline.
  b. Surgical decompression.

68.
  a. Rupture of the long head of biceps.
  b. Conservatively.

69.
  a. Gross striae atrophicae.
  b. Corticosteroid therapy.

70.
  a. Numerous fluid levels.
  b. Intestinal obstruction. The position and width of fluid levels differentiates small bowel from large bowel obstruction.

71.
  a. Eunuchoid proportions, absent body hair and small testes.
  b. Kallman's syndrome.

72.
  a. Oesophageal varices and oesophageal candidiasis.
  b. HIV serology.

73.
  a. Hyperlucency of the right lung.
  b. A foreign body, in this case a peanut, partially obstructing the right main bronchus.

74.
  a. Campbell De Morgan angiomas.
  b. Small bright red spots which occur on the trunk in the middle-aged and elderly and are of no clinical significance. They are often familial.

75.
a. Swelling and erythema over the fibrous flexor sheath of the index finger typical of a tendon sheath infection. Although there may be a preceding history, on occasions, no injury can be recalled.
b. Early antibiotic treatment is important, but if there is not a rapid return of normal finger movement surgical drainage and irrigation is important.

76.
a. A macular star due to hard exudates and cotton-wool spots.
b. Hypertension.

77.
a. Acute calcific tendonitis.
b. Treatment with analgesics and anti-inflammatory drugs. Aspiration or surgical removal of the calcium deposit will shorten the attack.

78.
a. Lupus vulgaris.
b. Anti-tuberculous chemotherapy.

79.
a. The two abnormalities illustrated are: discrete plane warts, and coalesced warts, illustrating the Koebner phenomenon.
b. The linear lesion, i.e. the Koebner phenomenon, occurred because of trauma.

80.
a. 'Tear drop' poikilocytosis.
b. Myelofibrosis.

81.
a. Endoscopic views of a large gastric ulcer containing blood clot indicating that this has been the site of bleeding.
b. Injection sclerotherapy with adrenaline to stop active bleeding followed by treatment with H_2 antagonists or omeprazole. Follow-up endoscopy is important to ensure healing of the ulcer and biopsies to exclude malignancy.

82.
a. Rheumatoid nodules around the elbow with overlying dermal infarcts.
b. Rheumatoid nodules indicate seropositive active rheumatoid disease.

83.
a. An Arnold–Chiari malformation.
b. It predisposes to hydrocephalus by obstructing the outlets of the fourth ventricle. The malformation is often associated with lumbosacral spina bifida.

84.
a. Normal fundus.

85.
a. Accelerated hypertension with arteriolar fibrinoid necrosis.
b. Retinal haemorrhage and papilloedema.

86.
a. Infection of the parafrenal (Tyson's) glands.
b. Gonococcus.
c. Urethral stricture.

87.
a. Left cervical rib.
b. Good oblique views should be obtained to visualize the intervertebral root exit foramina, CT scan either alone or in combination with myelography, NMR imaging, nerve conduction studies and EMG.

88.
a. Erythema marginatum.
b. Infection with *Streptococcus pyogenes*.

89.
a. Sudeck's osteodystrophy.
b. Failure to use an injured hand (in this case an undisplaced fracture of the distal radius) is a predisposing cause.

90.
a. ST elevation.
b. Pericarditis associated with chronic renal failure.

91.
a. White dermatographism.
b. The findings of no significance and the patients should be reassured.

92.
a. A subperichondrial haematoma.
b. The haematoma should be drained to prevent the development of fibrosis and cauliflower ear.

93.
a. Keratoderma blenorrhagica.
b. Reiter's syndrome. Associations include urethritis, back ache, calcaneal spurs, uncommonly pleurisy and pericarditis.

94.
a. Bilateral space-occupying lesions.
b. Bilateral acoustic neuromas.
c. Neurofibromatosis.

95.
a. A conjunctival melanoma.

96.
a. Paget's disease.
b. An increased plasma alkaline phosphatase of bony origin.
c. Complications other than bone fractures include nerve compression which may cause deafness or paraplegia, osteoarthritis, osteosarcoma, local pain and rarely high output cardiac failure.

97.
a. A classical Reed–Sternberg cell.
b. Hodgkin's disease; in this case of mixed cellularity type.

98.
a. A posterior central perforation of the eardrum.
b. The ear should be kept dry, and if recurrent otorrhoea occurs ear drops containing steroids and antibiotics should be used. A dry perforation can be repaired by myringoplasty. Traumatic central perforations usually heal spontaneously.

99.
a. Endoscopic retrograde cholangiopancreatography or ERCP.
b. A gallstone in the common bile duct.
c. This can frequently be removed endoscopically following sphincterotomy. In some cases, however, surgery is still necessary.

100.
a. Squamous cell carcinoma of the tongue.
b. Biopsy with histological confirmation.

101.
a. Bowen's disease.
b. It is strongly associated with internal malignancy.

102.
a. Papillary calcification with small kidneys.
b. Analgesic abuse.

103.
a. Hereditary haemorrhagic telangiectasia.
b. Cryosurgery or argon laser, if bleeding is troublesome. Also treat anaemia.

104.
a. Branch retinal artery occlusion.
b. Embolization from the internal carotids (e.g. platelet, cholesterol, calcium) or from the heart (mural thrombi, vegetations).

105.
a. Periarticular erosions in the foot.
b. Rheumatoid arthritis.

106.
a. Papulopustule of disseminated gonococcal infection.
b. Complications of disseminated gonococcal infections include arthropathy, a vasculitic rash and fever.

107.
a. Meningococcal septicaemia.
b. Treatment with benzylpenicillin and chloramphenicol.
c. Chemoprophylaxis for close contacts, such as people sharing a dormitory in the boarding school.

108.
a. A geographic tongue with areas of depapillation. These vary in size and distribution over a period of days.
b. No treatment is indicated other than that of the underlying condition.

109.
a. A ruptured Baker's cyst, which has become secondarily infected.
b. Rheumatoid arthritis.

110.
a. Seborrhoeic dermatitis.
b. This should be treated with soap substitutes and weak topical corticosteroids or corticosteroid-antibiotic combinations, tar shampoos, and sulphur and salicylic acid creams.

111.
a. A xeromammogram.
b. An area of increased fibrosis suggestive of breast carcinoma.

112.
a. An hepatic abscess causing a raised right hemidiaphragm and a fluid level.
b. Ultrasound needle aspiration or catheter insertion together with antibiotic treatment.

113.
a. Winging of the right scapula.
b. Damage to the long thoracic nerve (C5, 6, 7) either by trauma or by viral mononeuritis.

114.
a. A voiding cystourethrogram.
b. Reflux of contrast up the ureters on voiding.

115.
a. *Pneumocystis carinii* pneumonia.
b. Sputum, induced by inhalation of 3% nebulized saline, examined cytologically for pneumocysts, bronchoscopy and broncho-alveolar lavage with or without transbronchial biopsy.

116.
a. A pericardial effusion.
b. The pleural space and peritoneal cavity.

117.
a. Crohn's disease.
b. This should be treated like Crohn's elsewhere in the GI tract, with corticosteroids.

118.
a. A large bilateral mediastinal mass.
b. Hodgkin's disease.

119.
a. Swan-neck deformity.
b. Rheumatoid arthritis.

120.
a. A maculopapular rash.
b. This may occur shortly before seroconversion in HIV-infected individuals.

121.
a. Hypersensitivity skin tests to common allergens.
b. The multiple positive reaction suggests the subject is atopic.

122.
a. A calcaneal spur.
b. This is not an uncommon finding in asymptomatic people. However, it is associated with plantar fasciitis, and treatment with steroid injections, a heel pad or ultrasound therapy may be appropriate.

123.
a. Pre-proliferative diabetic retinopathy characterized by venous dilatation and irregularities, cotton-wool spots, intraretinal shunts and attenuated arterioles.
b. Diabetes mellitus.
c. Good metabolic control and regular eye examination. Photocoagulation is indicated for proliferative retinopathy and certain maculopathies.

124.
a. Porphyria cutanea tarda.
b. Alcoholic liver disease, chronic hepatitis C virus infection and hepatocellular carcinoma.

125.
a. 'Tram-line' shadowing.
b. Bronchiectasis.

126.
a. Koilonychia.
b. It may be associated with chronic iron-deficiency anaemia.

127.
a. Neurofibromatosis affecting both hands.
b. Other abnormalities include: abnormal pigmentation of the skin, skeletal deformity and soft tissue tumours; acoustic neuromas and phaeochromocytomas are also associated.
c. Autosomal dominant inheritance.

128.
a. Nephrocalcinosis.
b. Renal tubular acidosis.

129.
a. Lichen planus.
b. Treatment should be with topical corticosteroids either as cream or ointment.

130.
a. Periostitis of the tibiae and fibulae.
b. Hypertrophic pulmonary osteoarthropathy. Most often associated with bronchogenic carcinoma.

131.
a. A Meckel's diverticulum.
b. Bleeding is due to ulceration of ectopic gastric epithelium within the diverticulum.

132.
a. A tattoo, an abscess and needle track inflammation.
b. Hepatitis B and C, and HIV infection.

133.
a. Chronic uveitis with keratic precipitates.
b. With corticosteroids.

134.
a. A giant-cell tumour of the distal radius.
b. Excision if possible. Local recurrence may occur if excision is incomplete. Metastatic spread however, is rare.

135.
a. Septicaemia, probably gonococcal.
b. Investigations include blood culture and culture of material from the peripheral spots if available.

136.
a. Segmental retinopathy with areas of exudation and haemorrhage.
b. Cytomegalovirus (CMV) retinitis.

137.
a. Acquired ichthyosis.
b. The most common underlying cause is a lymphoproliferative

disorder such as Hodgkin's disease or mycosis fungoides.
Less common causes are malabsorption, malnutrition or
drug reaction.

138.
a. Three duodenal ulcers.
b. A serum gastrin concentration.

139.
a. Nail hypoplasia as part of the nail-patella syndrome.
b. Other skeletal deformities include absence of the patellae,
bony abnormalities of the elbows, and ilial spurs.

140.
a. Legionnaire's disease.
b. Early diagnosis may be obtained by specific antigen
detection in urine or bronchial brushings and washings.
Serological tests of antibody production are useful in
confirming the diagnosis, but may only appear later in the
illness.

141.
a. Ankle oedema and yellowish discolouration of the nails.
b. The yellow nail syndrome, which is made up of congenital
bronchiectasis, lymphoedema and yellow discolouration of
the nails.

142.
a. Ossification of the intervertebral ligaments giving rise to a
'bamboo spine' appearance.
b. Anterior uveitis, aortic regurgitation, apical pulmonary
fibrosis, myopathy and amyloidosis.

143.
a. Pyoderma gangrenosum.
b. This is usually associated with ulcerative colitis and Crohn's
disease. Collagen vascular diseases, blood dyscrasias,
lymphomas and sarcoidosis are occasional causes and no
cause is found in 20% of cases.

144.
a. Angiodysplasia in the colon.
b. Patient admitted because of rectal bleeding and anaemia.
There is also an association with aortic stenosis.

145.
a. This is superficial inflammatory acne.
b. Important aetiological factors include genetic, androgens,
abnormal sebum production, colonization of the
pylosebaceous unit with *Propionibacterium acnes*, obstruction
of the sebaceous duct and inflammation.

146.
a. Tinea corporis.
b. Treatment should be with topical antifungal agents,
e.g. imidazole cream or oral terbinafine for 4–5 weeks.

147.
a. Osteomyelitis of the lower end of the tibia.
b. Blood cultures to identify the infecting organism, X-rays to

look for subperiosteal reaction although these may initially be negative and an isotope bone scan to look for increased uptake over the area.

148.
a. Crohn's disease.
b. Biopsies for histological confirmation.

149.
a. A lung abscess with an air-fluid level.
b. Lung abscesses complicate aspiration pneumonia, pulmonary infarction and septic embolization.

150.
a. Molluscum contagiosum.
b. Immunosuppression, particularly AIDS.

151.
a. This is an examination being undertaken under Wood's light.
b. The characteristic green/blue fluorescence is typical of tinea capitis or ringworm.

152.
a. Condylomata lata.
b. Acquired secondary syphilis.
c. Penicillin is the treatment of choice, with tetracyclines or erythromycin as alternatives in individuals with penicillin hypersensitivity.

153.
a. Livedo reticularis.
b. This is associated with polyarteritis nodosa and systemic lupus erythematosus.

154.
a. Disseminated Kaposi's sarcoma.
b. HIV infection.
c. It indicates AIDS.

155.
a. Retroperitoneal haemorrhage.
b. Acute haemorrhagic pancreatitis.

156.
a. Rubella.
b. Lymphadenopathy, especially suboccipital and post auricular, is common.

157.
a. Oesophageal web.
b. This may be associated with iron deficiency anaemia in women as part of the Plummer–Vinson or Patterson–Brown–Kelly syndrome.

158.
a. This is guttate psoriasis, illustrating rain-drop lesions.
b. Guttate psoriasis is commoner in the young and may be precipitated by a streptococcal sore throat.

159.
a. Psoriasis and onycholysis.
b. Fungal infection and eczema.

160.
a. An 'hair-on-end' appearance.
b. Thalassaemia.

161.
a. Leukoplakia of the tongue.
b. This may complicate any cause of chronic glossitis such as smoking, syphilis or betel chewing. Most instances are of unknown cause.

162.
a. Acute ethmoiditis with orbital cellulitis.
b. This is an emergency and patients should be admitted to hospital, antibiotics started and the maxillary sinuses washed out if also infected. A CT scan should be performed if the possibility of an orbital abscess is considered.

163.
a. Lupus pernio.
b. This is associated with sarcoidosis.
c. Treatment with oral corticosteroids in the presence of systemic symptoms.

164.
a. Prolapse has occurred around the stoma resulting in it lying flush with the skin.
b. This has resulted in leakage of stomal contents on the skin resulting in irritation which has been treated by the patient with a steroid cream resulting in skin atrophy.

165.
a. Hypercholesterolaemia leading to cutaneous xanthomata and perineural lipid deposits.
b. Plasmapheresis.

166.
a. Toxic epidermal necrosis.
b. Immunosuppression increases the risk of staphylococcal infection.

167.
a. Urinary calculus in the line of the left ureter.
b. Serum and urinary calcium and urate, renal ultrasound and IVU; if indicated, urine cystine.

168.
a. Acne rosacea.
b. This should be treated by avoiding exacerbating factors such as the sun, heat, alcohol, hot/spicy foods, and by giving low-dose antibiotics (e.g. oxytetracycline) for months or years.

169.
a. Bilateral singer's nodules.
b. In this particular case, his job as an auctioneer is probably important and voice rest should be advocated. Speech therapy may also play a role. Endoscopic removal should also be considered.

170.
a. A large spider naevus.
b. The presence of four or more spider naevi or less if they are

large should suggest underlying cirrhosis. They may also occur in the third trimester of pregnancy, remitting after delivery, and in rheumatoid arthritis.

171.
a. A white strawberry tongue with circumoral pallor.
b. Scarlet fever.

172.
a. Seborrhoeic wart.
b. This lesion, which should be differentiated from malignant melanoma or a pigmented basal cell carcinoma, can be treated simply by curettage or cryotherapy.

173.
a. Ankylosing spondylitis with bilateral sacroiliitis and symphyseal arthritis.
b. HLA antigen status, looking specifically for HLA B27.

174.
a. A thoracotomy scar with surrounding nodules due to mesothelioma.
b. Asbestosis.

175.
a. Milroy's disease.
b. Congenital abnormality in the lymphatics of the lower or upper limb. This causes chronic non-pitting oedema. Associated problems include pleural effusions and chylous ascites.

176.
a. Fibro-muscular dysplasia with typical 'beaded' appearance of the renal arteries.
b. Between 1–5%.

177.
a. Oral thrush.
b. Altered oral ecology due to antibiotics, corticosteroids, xerostomia, diabetes mellitus, or immune defects (e.g. AIDS, immunosuppressive treatment, leukaemia, lymphoma).

178.
a. Atypical mononuclear cells.
b. Infectious mononucleosis or glandular fever.

179.
a. This picture illustrates cutis laxa, a characteristic feature of Ehlers–Danlos syndrome.
b. Other features that should be looked for include hypermobile or hyperextensible joints, fragile skin with easy bruising, wide atrophic scars, and blue sclera.

180.
a. A keratoacanthoma.
b. These do not require treatment as they will resolve spontaneously.

181.
a. Gold treatment.
b. Withdrawal of gold leads to slow clearing of the rash.

182.
a. An Osler's node.
b. Infective endocarditis.

183.
a. Hemiatrophy of the right side of the tongue.
b. Lower motor neuron lesion of the right twelfth cranial nerve.

184.
a. Ulnar deviation of the fingers of the right hand, and pronounced palmar erythema.
b. Palmar erythema is associated with cirrhosis, especially alcoholic cirrhosis.

185.
a. This radiograph shows pancreatic calcification and opaque gall stones.
b. Ultrasound or CT scanning and an ERCP.

186.
a. This is necrobiosis lipidoica which usually affects the front of the shins.
b. The most likely underlying diagnosis is diabetes mellitus.

187.
a. Horner's syndrome affecting the right eye.
b. An apical bronchogenic carcinoma.

188.
a. Gingival swelling.
b. Acute monocytic leukaemia.
c. Full blood count and film.

189.
a. Secondary syphilis.
b. Serological confirmation including TPHA and ELISA for anti-treponemal IgM.

190.
a. This is a barium enema showing features typical of an intussusception.
b. Although in children this may be reduced by the barium enema investigation, in adults it usually requires surgery.

191.
a. Bilateral antral fluid levels.
b. Treatment is with antibiotics, and antral washout if resolution is not rapid.

192.
a. Enlarged sulci of cortical atrophy.
b. AIDS dementia syndrome.

193.
a. Dermatitis artefacta.
b. The lesion should be kept occluded, for example with a plastercast, and psychiatric help sought.

194.
a. A percutaneous transhepatic cholangiogram.
b. Sclerosing cholangitis.

195.
a. Proptosis with pronounced vascular injection.
b. A carotico-cavernous fistula.

196.
a. Macular pigmentation of fingertips in Peutz-Jeghers syndrome.
b. Perioral lentiginosis.
c. Small intestinal polyps.

197.
a. Acute orf.
b. The lesion heals spontaneously over several weeks and no specific treatment is available. It should not be incised. Erythromycin or flucloxacillin are effective for secondary bacterial infection.

198.
a. Bilateral hydronephrosis.
b. Bladder, cervical or prostatic tumours, retroperitoneal fibrosis, spinal cord lesions, urethral valves.

199.
a. Xanthelasma.
b. Primary biliary cirrhosis.

200.
a. A glomus tumour under the thumb nail.
b. Adequate excision, as recurrence will occur if the whole tumour is not removed.

201.
a. Chronic osteomyelitis of the tibia.
b. Renal amyloidosis.

202.
a. Anterior mediastinal mass due to a thymoma.
b. Acquired red cell aplasia may be associated with a thymoma causing severe anaemia. Myaesthenia gravis may be associated with thymoma causing these symptoms.

203.
a. Oesophageal varices.
b. An upper gastrointestinal endoscopy should be undertaken to confirm that the varices were the site of bleeding and if so injection sclerotherapy or band ligation should be performed until the varices are eradicated.

204.
a. Fine wrinkled skin with thinning hair.
b. Hypopituitarism.

205.
a. Spondylolisthesis between L5 and S1.
b. Surgical fusion of the appropriate spinal segments is appropriate for symptoms in younger patients.

206.
a. An eschar.
b. Anthrax.

207.
a. This is tinea pedis or atheletes' foot due to tinea or ringworm infections. This appearance may also be caused by bacteria, candida or sweating.

b. Should be treated with topical antifungal agents such as imidazole cream. For more extensive infections, oral terbinafine may be necessary.

208.
a. Pseudomembranous colitis.
b. Treatment is usually with vancomycin.

209.
a. Nodular fibromas.
b. Phaeochromocytoma and hyperparathyroidism as part of multiple endocrine adenoma syndrome type II (Sipple's syndrome).

210.
a. A large vascular naevus on the left side of the face.
b. Sturge–Weber syndrome.
c. Cerebral calcification and focal atrophy are common and predispose to epilepsy.

211.
a. Splinter haemorrhages.
b. Infective endocarditis.
c. Most likely cause is immune complex glomerulonephritis.

212.
a. Invasive pulmonary aspergillosis.
b. Immunosuppression with steroid treatment predisposes to systemic involvement with fungal septicaemia. It should be treated with systemic anti-fungal therapy, e.g. amphotericin.

213.
a. Finger clubbing and skin pigmentation.
b. Primary biliary cirrhosis.

214.
a. The most likely cause for generalized excoriations are body lice (pediculosis corporis).
b. Should be treated by improved hygiene, thorough disinfection of clothing, and 0.5% carbaryl/0.5% malathion lotions.

215.
a. A large blister on the left wrist.
b. Self poisoning with barbiturates.

216.
a. Retinitis proliferans.
b. Retinal haemorrhage or fibrous contraction resulting in retinal detachment.

217.
a. Addison's disease.
b. Pigmentation may also be found in the buccal cavity, the lips and areas of solar exposure.

218.
a. Pathological fracture of the humerus due to metastatic tumour.
b. If the site of the primary tumour is not obvious a biopsy from the fracture site will provide histological confirmation of tumour type.

219.
a. Diabetes mellitus.
b. Factors involved in ulcer formation include neuropathy resulting in diminished pain sensation, secondary infection, and ischaemia.

220.
a. Acanthosis nigricans.
b. It is often associated with underlying malignancy.

221.
a. A caput medusae.
b. Portal hypertension.
c. Bleeding is probably due to oesophageal varices, which should be treated with endoscopic injection sclerotherapy, at least initially.

222.
a. Synovial chondromatosis forming loose bodies within the knee joint.
b. Surgical removal of loose bodies and synovectomy.

223.
a. Leukoplakia.
b. It is premalignant.

224.
a. Allergic contact dermatitis.
b. Allergy due to nickel jean stud. This is a type IV (delayed) lymphocyte-mediated hypersensitivity. Other common allergens include rubber, chromate and cosmetics.

225.
a. Bullous lesions and mucosal ulceration.
b. The likely diagnosis of Stevens-Johnson syndrome may be caused by hypersensitivity to drugs such as sulphonamides and penicillins, or by infections due to herpes simplex, *Mycoplasma pneumoniae* and streptococci.

226.
a. A black hairy tongue.
b. This condition is asymptomatic although the appearance may upset the patient. Treatment is by mechanical brushing or scraping of the dorsum of the tongue.

227.
a. This shows a bone infarct in the medulla of the femur.
b. This is often asymptomatic, but if adjacent to a joint loss of support of the nearby articular cartilage may result in joint deformity and secondary osteoarthritis.

228.
a. Multiple polypoid filling defects throughout the colon.
b. Familial adenomatous polyposis.

229.
a. A subconjunctival haemorrhage.
b. Pertussis (whooping cough).

230.
a. This demonstrates the stacked penny sign.
b. Systemic sclerosis or scleroderma.

231.
a. Calcification of the lateral meniscus of the knee.
b. Chondrocalcinosis (pseudogout).

232.
a. Hereditary angioedema.
b. Acute attacks should be treated by injection of C1 esterase inhibitor or infusion of fresh frozen plasma. Severe attacks may require subcutaneous adrenaline (1:1000) injection. Preventative treatment: stanozolol, tranexamic acid, danazol for hereditary angioedema.
c. Deficiency of C1 esterase inhibitor.

233.
a. Scrotal ulcers.
b. Behçet's syndrome.

234.
a. Bilateral hilar lymphadenopathy compressing the right upper lobe bronchus.
b. Lymphoma and sarcoidosis are the two main diagnoses to exclude.

235.
a. Onycholysis.
b. Causes include: trauma, infection, psoriasis, dermatitis, ischaemia, drug reaction, and thyroid disease.

236.
a. Granuloma annulare.
b. In adults, approximately one-third of patients with granuloma annulare have diabetes mellitus or abnormal glucose tolerance.

237.
a. Beau's lines.
b. The lines are caused by interruption of nail-bed growth during severe illness and are seen weeks later when nail growth has recommenced.

238.
a. Atrophic glossitis with angular stomatitis.
b. Vitamin B deficiency should be excluded.

239.
a. This illustrates flaccid blisters and erosions typical of pemphigus.
b. Firm lateral pressure is put on the skin surface with the thumb. The epidermis appears to slide over the underlying dermis, i.e. Nikolsky's sign.

240.
a. Multiple filling defects in the liver typical of metastatic disease.
b. Ultrasound or CT-guided liver biopsy, alphafetoprotein, chest X-ray, barium enema, depending upon likely site of the primary tumour.

241.
a. A 'pepper-pot' skull with multiple lytic lesions.
b. Myelomatosis.

c. Identification of a paraprotein band on electrophoresis, and Bence-Jones proteinuria due to light chains (not detected by dip-stix), and bone-marrow aspiration revealing a plasma-cell infiltrate.

242. a. Eczema due to venous stasis, 'atrophie blanche'.
b. Venous hypertension due to deep vein thrombosis or from familial valvular incompetence.

243. a. A lingual thyroid.
b. Functioning thyroid tissue should be identified in the neck before the lingual thyroid mass is removed, otherwise hypothroidism will develop.

244. a. Long slender fingers.
b. Marfan's syndrome. The general laxity of connective tissue may cause dislocation of lenses of the eye as well as aortic dilatation and incompetence.

245. a. Early slip of the left femoral epiphysis.
b. Avascular necrosis with loss of articular cartilage and deformity causing secondary osteoarthritis.

246. a. Frostbite of the fingertips.
b. In the acute phase, the whole patient should be warmed and low-molecular-weight dextran given intravenously. Amputation should be delayed until there is a clear line of demarcation between viable and nonviable tissue.

247. a. Localized morphoea.
b. This is a localized cutaneous form of scleroderma or progressive systemic sclerosis.

248. a. Widespread haemorrhages and retinal infarcts with blurring of the optic disc margin.
b. Megaloblastic anaemia.

249. a. Periungal fibroma.
b. Tuberous sclerosis.

250. a. A chicken bone in the hypopharynx.
b. Complications include airways oedema, soft tissue infection or oesophageal perforation.

251. a. Strawberry naevus.
b. No treatment is required, as the lesions spontaneously resolve.

252. a. Left facial weakness due to Bell's palsy.
b. Cranial neuropathy in patients with stage IV AIDS.

253.
a. Adult respiratory distress syndrome.
b. Typically, there is hypoxia with a normal or mildly elevated $PaCO_2$ and frequently a metabolic acidosis.

254.
a. Lichen simplex (neurodermatitis), which is a localized eruption developing in response to constant rubbing, often due to habit and/or stress.
b. Treatment should be with potent topical steroids, tar and sedative antihistamines.

255.
a. Right third nerve palsy.
b. Diabetic mononeuritis.

256.
a. Gonorrhoea.
b. The diagnosis must be confirmed by culture on selective media such as MNYC in a CO_2-enriched atmosphere with identification of suspected colonies by oxidase reaction, sugar utilization tests, coagglutination and immunofluorescence.

257.
a. Perifollicular haemorrhages in scurvy. This is usually most obvious on the lower limbs.
b. It should be treated with oral vitamin C; other manifestations include spontaneous haemorrhage and bleeding from the gums.

258.
a. A barium enema showing faecal impaction.
b. Hirschsprung's disease.

Index